Pediatric Endocrinology – Advances in Diagnosis and Treatment

Edited by Robert Gensure

Published in London, United Kingdom

Pediatric Endocrinology - Advances in Diagnosis and Treatment
http://dx.doi.org/10.5772/intechopen.1009049
Edited by Robert Gensure

Contributors
Abdullah M. Assiri, Amna Mohammed Idris Musa, Aylin Kılınç Uğurlu, Aymen Nasreldin Abdalkariem Mohammed, Cynthia Ruiz-Carranza, Elizabeth E. Littlejohn, Harrison Samuel, Helen Harrison, Irasema Apodaca-Ramos, Itedal Abdelraheem Mohamed Ahmed, Khlood M. Mehdar, Mishkat Hatim Ali Khalil, Mohammed Ayed Huneif

First published in London, United Kingdom, 2026 by IntechOpen
IntechOpen is the global imprint of INTECHOPEN LIMITED, registered in England and Wales, registration number: 11086078, 167-169 Great Portland Street, London, W1W 5PF, United Kingdom

For EU product safety concerns: IN TECH d.o.o., Prolaz Marije Krucifikse Kozulić 3, 51000 Rijeka, Croatia, info@intechopen.com or visit our website at intechopen.com.

British Library Cataloguing-in-Publication Data
A catalogue record for this book is available from the British Library

Pediatric Endocrinology - Advances in Diagnosis and Treatment
Edited by Robert Gensure
p. cm.
Print ISBN 978-1-83769-928-5
Online ISBN 978-1-83769-927-8
eBook (PDF) ISBN 978-1-83769-929-2

If disposing of this product, please recycle the paper responsibly.

Meet the editor

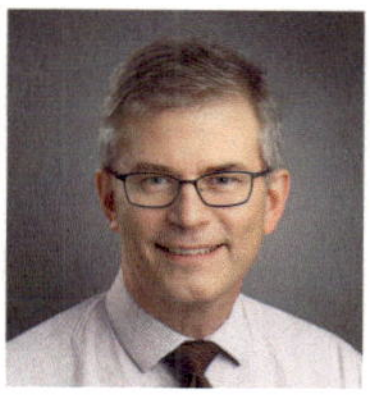

Robert Gensure, MD, Ph.D., is a physician-scientist with significant experience in basic science and clinical research as well as in the clinical practice of pediatric endocrinology. He has authored over 60 publications on topics including parathyroid hormone, parathyroid hormone-related peptide, vitamin D supplementation, alopecia, and inherited disorders of bone and mineral metabolism. He is currently the chief of pediatric endocrinology at Dartmouth Health Children's in NH, US.

Contents

Preface

There have been significant advances in pediatric endocrinology, particularly in diabetes and weight management. Research in weight management has elucidated the causes of pediatric obesity, and there are now several therapeutic options to assist with weight control. Increasingly, pediatric endocrinologists are providing medical therapy for obesity in place of bariatric surgery. GLP-1 agonists lead the field in these areas, but there are other therapeutic options to consider when managing patients with weight disorders. In addition to providing treatment for pediatric obesity, pediatric endocrinologists continue to provide supportive roles for comprehensive weight programs, managing comorbid conditions such as PCOS and type 2 diabetes mellitus. This book provides a comprehensive review of these new areas of pediatric endocrine practice and is a critical resource for ensuring that the latest care recommendations are followed.

There have also been significant advances in the management of type 1 diabetes mellitus. We can now more clearly distinguish type 1 diabetes from other related disorders, such as Maturity-Onset Diabetes of the Young, which have distinct pathogenesis and therapies. There is a growing understanding of how diabetes develops in children, and research into strategies to prevent or postpone this progression. Most importantly, there have been significant advances in diabetes management technology. Insulin pumps are now integrated with continuous glucose monitors and use artificial intelligence-enhanced algorithms to provide limited closed-loop features to autoregulate blood sugar. These algorithms can adapt as children's insulin needs change with growth and development. The role of the endocrinologist is gradually shifting towards assisting patients in optimally utilizing these new tools, which allow children greater freedom in living with diabetes. Diets have become much less restrictive, and children can pursue a broader range of activities. These advances have a direct impact on the practice of pediatric endocrinology. The book reviews these developments and how practice standards are evolving in response to them.

Our understanding of disorders of the pituitary gland has been significantly enhanced by research into their genetic basis. We are now better able to classify pituitary disorders, with enhanced ability to predict prognosis and to tailor therapies for individual patients. The physiology of the pituitary gland and the management of pituitary hormone deficiencies are reviewed extensively in this book. Lastly, there is a discussion of interactions of hormone systems, specifically on vitamin D and thyroid function.

Overall, the book provides important information and updates on areas critical to the future of pediatric endocrinology and offers tools to help practitioners deliver optimal care for patients in these areas.

Robert Gensure, M.D./Ph.D.
Chief,
Pediatric Endocrinology,
Dartmouth Health Children's
Lebanon, NH, USA

Associate Professor,
Geisel School of Medicine at Dartmouth,
Lebanon, NH, USA

Section 1

Diabetes Mellitus

Chapter 1

Type 1 Diabetes Mellitus

Aylin Kılınç Uğurlu

Abstract

Type 1 diabetes mellitus (T1DM) is the most common chronic endocrine disorder of childhood and is increasing worldwide. It is defined by immune-mediated destruction of pancreatic β-cells in genetically susceptible individuals – principally those carrying HLA-DR3/DR4-DQ2/DQ8 haplotypes – with additional contributions from non-HLA loci (e.g., INS, PTPN22, CTLA4, IL2RA) and environmental triggers such as viral infections, early-life nutritional exposures, vitamin D deficiency, microbiome dysbiosis, and obesity-related insulin resistance. The disease often presents abruptly after ~80%–90% β-cell loss with polyuria, polydipsia, weight loss, and, in 20%–40% of cases, diabetic ketoacidosis. Diagnosis relies on ADA/ISPAD glucose or HbA1c thresholds, supported by islet autoantibodies and preserved C-peptide patterns in differential diagnoses. Management centers on lifelong insulin replacement delivered as multiple daily injections or continuous subcutaneous insulin infusion, increasingly optimized by continuous glucose monitoring and hybrid closed-loop systems. Individualized glycemic targets (HbA1c < 7.0% for most; CGM time-in-range > 70%) balance safety and efficacy across developmental stages. Acute complications include hypoglycemia and DKA; chronic complications warrant structured screening for retinopathy, nephropathy, neuropathy, dyslipidemia, and hypertension, alongside surveillance for associated autoimmune diseases. Preventive strategies now include risk stratification by autoantibodies and emerging immunotherapies; notably, teplizumab delays progression from stage 2 to clinical T1DM. Comprehensive, multidisciplinary care remains essential to optimize outcomes.

Keywords: type 1 diabetes mellitus, children, diagnosis, continuous glucose monitoring system, management

1. Introduction

Diabetes mellitus (DM) is a chronic endocrine and metabolic disorder characterized by hyperglycemia resulting from impaired insulin secretion and/or action. Insulin, synthesized by the pancreatic beta cells, regulates energy homeostasis. Inadequate insulin release and/or reduced tissue responsiveness to insulin impair its biological effects in target tissues, leading to disturbances in carbohydrate, lipid, and protein metabolism [1]. Type 1 diabetes (T1D) mellitus (T1DM) is a chronic metabolic disease commonly observed in childhood, caused by the destruction of pancreatic beta cells, resulting in absolute insulin deficiency. T1DM accounts for more than 90% of pediatric diabetes cases [2].

T1DM is not solely a metabolic disorder but a lifelong condition that profoundly impacts both the individual and the family. Treatment extends beyond insulin replacement to include structured education, utilization of technological tools, psychosocial support, and early detection of complications.

The significance of the disease arises not only from its high prevalence but also from the risk of complications. Poor metabolic control leads to the development of microvascular complications (retinopathy, nephropathy, neuropathy) and, in the long term, macrovascular complications.

The benefits of intensive insulin therapy were demonstrated by the Diabetes Control and Complications Trial (DCCT), which showed that patients receiving intensive therapy had a 50%–76% lower risk of retinopathy, nephropathy, and neuropathy [3, 4]. The long-term follow-up study, EDIC (Epidemiology of Diabetes Interventions and Complications), further revealed that early achievement of good glycemic control is associated with reduced cardiovascular events [4].

In recent years, groundbreaking advances have been made in diabetes care. Continuous glucose monitoring (CGM) systems, insulin pumps, and hybrid closed-loop systems (AID) have significantly improved glycemic outcomes in children and adolescents [5]. Furthermore, teplizumab has emerged as the first immunomodulatory therapy approved by the FDA to delay progression to clinical-stage T1DM, highlighting the potential to alter the natural history of the disease [6, 7].

2. Definition and classification

DM is a heterogeneous group of metabolic disorders characterized by chronic hyperglycemia resulting from impaired insulin secretion, defective insulin action, or a combination of both, leading to disturbances in carbohydrate, lipid, and protein metabolism. This definition encompasses T1D (absolute insulin deficiency due to autoimmune β-cell destruction), type 2 diabetes (relative insulin secretory defect combined with insulin resistance), monogenic forms of diabetes (MODY, neonatal diabetes), and secondary diabetes (resulting from pancreatic diseases, endocrinopathies, or drug-induced causes) [1].

The most common form of diabetes in childhood is T1D. In the autoimmune form of T1D, autoantibodies against islet antigens (GAD65, IA-2A, ZnT8A, and insulin autoantibodies) are detected. This autoimmune response leads to T cell–mediated β-cell destruction, culminating in absolute insulin deficiency [8]. The clinical onset is typically abrupt; children are usually lean or of normal weight and present with polyuria, polydipsia, and weight loss. At diagnosis, the likelihood of diabetic ketoacidosis (DKA) is high [9]. This form is currently defined as type 1A diabetes. The rarer form, type 1B or idiopathic T1D, is characterized by the absence of autoantibodies, occurs more frequently in individuals of African or Asian origin, and is often associated with a strong tendency toward ketosis. In some cases, both autoimmunity and obesity-related insulin resistance coexist; this phenotype is referred to as "double diabetes" [10].

Type 2 diabetes is increasingly recognized in the pediatric age group. It typically arises in genetically predisposed adolescents in association with obesity and insulin resistance. Clinical features often include abdominal obesity, acanthosis nigricans, and a family history of type 2 diabetes. DKA is less common at presentation, though hyperosmolar hyperglycemic syndrome (HHS) may occur. Laboratory findings generally reveal negative autoantibodies, normal or elevated C-peptide concentrations, and frequent coexistence of dyslipidemia and hepatic steatosis [11].

Monogenic forms of diabetes result from single-gene mutations and are often misdiagnosed as T1D. The best-known subgroup is Maturity-Onset Diabetes of the Young (MODY). MODY2, caused by glucokinase mutations, is characterized by mild and stable fasting hyperglycemia and generally does not require pharmacological treatment. MODY due to HNF1A or HNF4A mutations leads to progressive hyperglycemia; patients show remarkable sensitivity to low-dose sulfonylureas. HNF1B mutations are associated not only with diabetes but also with renal cysts and structural renal anomalies; most affected individuals require insulin therapy [12]. Neonatal diabetes, a distinct monogenic entity presenting within the first six months of life, may be transient or permanent. Transient neonatal diabetes is most commonly linked to genetic abnormalities at chromosome 6q24 and may remit in infancy but relapse during adolescence. Permanent neonatal diabetes most often results from KCNJ11 or ABCC8 mutations, with many patients responding successfully to high-dose sulfonylurea therapy [13]. Other monogenic forms include mitochondrial diabetes (MIDD), diabetes associated with insulin receptor defects, and lipodystrophy-related diabetes[12].

Secondary diabetes arises in the context of other diseases or treatments. The most prominent example is cystic fibrosis–related diabetes (CFRD), caused by a combination of exocrine pancreatic insufficiency and β-cell dysfunction; oral glucose tolerance testing (OGTT) screening is recommended from the age of 10 years [14]. Chronic pancreatitis, pancreatectomy, or pancreatic tumors may also lead to diabetes. Among endocrinopathies, Cushing syndrome, acromegaly, hyperthyroidism, pheochromocytoma, and glucagonoma are associated with hyperglycemia. Moreover, various medications, including glucocorticoids, tacrolimus, cyclosporine, sirolimus, L-asparaginase, atypical antipsychotics, and protease inhibitors, can induce diabetes. Post-transplant diabetes, related to immunosuppressive therapy after solid organ transplantation, also belongs to this category [15].

3. Epidemiology

T1DM incidence is steadily increasing worldwide. The global incidence and prevalence of T1DM vary considerably across countries.

According to data from 2024, an estimated 1.81 million children and adolescents (<20 years of age) were living with T1D worldwide. In the same year, 219,000 new cases of T1D were diagnosed among individuals under 20 years of age [16].

The highest incidence rates have been reported in Northern European countries, particularly Finland and Sweden, which rank among the nations with the highest burden of T1DM worldwide. In Finland, the incidence reaches 60–65 per 100,000 child-years, while in Sweden, it is approximately 45–50 per 100,000 child-years. These figures are several-fold higher than the global average, placing these countries in the "high-incidence regions." Other European countries with similarly high rates include Iceland, Norway, and the United Kingdom. Intermediate-incidence countries include Germany, the Netherlands, Canada, Australia, and the United States, where reported annual incidence typically ranges from 15 to 30 per 100,000 child-years. Turkey, similar to other Mediterranean countries, falls within the intermediate-incidence category, with recent data indicating an incidence of approximately 20 per 100,000 child-years in children and adolescents. By contrast, low-incidence regions are represented primarily by Asian and African countries. In populous nations such as China, India, Japan, and Korea, the annual incidence of T1DM is only 1–5 per 100,000 child-years. Similarly, most African countries report incidence rates below 5 per 100,000 child-years. In these settings, environmental factors, in addition to genetic susceptibility, are considered to play a critical role. Overall, T1DM demonstrates nearly a 20-fold variation in incidence between the highest-risk Scandinavian countries and the lowest-risk regions of Asia and Africa. This disparity underscores the contribution of both genetic predisposition and environmental/lifestyle factors in shaping the epidemiology of the disease [15].

A notable trend in recent years has been the shift toward earlier onset of T1DM. Although incidence previously peaked between ages 10 and 14 years, a significant increase is now observed among children under 5 years of age. As this phenomenon cannot be explained solely by genetics, environmental exposures – such as early-life feeding practices, viral infections, vitamin D status, and alterations in the gut microbiome – are believed to play a major role [17]. Importantly, earlier onset complicates the achievement of optimal metabolic control and places an additional burden on family quality of life.

4. Pathogenesis

The pathogenesis of T1DM is a complex process initiated by environmental triggers in genetically susceptible individuals, culminating in immune-mediated destruction of pancreatic β-cells. The disease is multifactorial, with strong interactions among genetic, environmental, and immunological components.

T1DM is a polygenic disease, with genetic predisposition forming the cornerstone of susceptibility. Among these, HLA class II genes represent the strongest risk factors, particularly haplotypes HLA-DR3, DR4, DQ2, and DQ8, which markedly increase disease risk [17]. Individuals carrying these genotypes face a lifetime risk of developing diabetes as high as 20%, compared with ~0.4% in the general population. In first-degree relatives of affected patients, the risk rises to approximately 1.3–9%. Monozygotic twin concordance rates of 30%–50% highlight that genetic predisposition alone is insufficient, and environmental factors also contribute substantially. Beyond HLA, several non-HLA genes contribute to disease risk, including INS (insulin VNTR polymorphisms), PTPN22 (protein tyrosine phosphatase non-receptor type 22), CTLA4 (cytotoxic T-lymphocyte–associated antigen 4), and IL2RA (interleukin-2 receptor α). These genes influence immune tolerance and T-cell regulation, facilitating initiation of the autoimmune process. Currently, polygenic risk scores incorporating these loci are used to identify high-risk individuals [15].

Environmental factors are considered key triggers of the autoimmune cascade in genetically predisposed individuals. Viral infections – particularly enteroviruses – have been implicated, exerting either direct cytotoxic effects on β-cells or initiating molecular mimicry that provokes autoimmunity. Early nutritional exposures, such as cow's milk protein and gluten, have been investigated as potential risk modifiers, though findings remain inconsistent. Vitamin D deficiency, given its immunomodulatory role, has been associated with increased T1DM risk. Dysbiosis of the gut microbiota and early-life antibiotic use may further disrupt immune tolerance. In addition, childhood obesity and rapid growth, by inducing insulin resistance, may accelerate β-cell stress and disease progression [18].

The immunological process lies at the core of T1DM. The disease is characterized by both humoral and cellular immune responses against islet autoantigens. Islet autoantibodies (GAD65, IA-2A, insulin autoantibodies, ZnT8A) are detectable years before clinical diabetes (stage 3b), serving as diagnostic markers. However, the principal mediators of β-cell destruction are T lymphocytes. CD8 + cytotoxic T cells directly target β-cells, while CD4 + helper T cells amplify inflammation through cytokine production (In't Veld, *Diabetes* 2011). Pro-inflammatory cytokines such as IFN-γ, IL-1β, and TNF-α induce β-cell apoptosis and exacerbate the autoimmune cascade.

The natural history of T1DM has been staged [7].

- **Stage 1**: Multiple autoantibody positivity with normoglycemia.
- **Stage 2**: Dysglycemia develops, characterized by impaired fasting glucose, abnormal OGTT, or rising HbA1c.
- **Stage 3a**: Asymptomatic hyperglycemia.
- **Stage 3b**: Symptomatic clinical diabetes with polyuria, polydipsia, weight loss, or DKA.
- **Stage 4**: Long-standing diabetes, where chronic complications emerge.

Recently, immunomodulatory therapies have demonstrated the potential to alter the natural history of T1DM. The anti-CD3 monoclonal antibody teplizumab delayed progression to clinical diabetes by an average of two years in high-risk individuals with multiple autoantibodies and dysglycemia [7]. This finding shifts the paradigm from treating T1DM only at its symptomatic stage toward the possibility of preventive interventions.

5. Clinical features and diagnosis

The clinical presentation of T1DM typically emerges once approximately 80%–90% of pancreatic β-cell mass has been lost. Beyond this threshold, insulin secretion becomes insufficient to maintain normoglycemia, leading to overt hyperglycemia and the appearance of symptoms.

The classic triad consists of polyuria, polydipsia, polyphagia, and weight loss. Polyuria results from hyperglycemia exceeding the renal threshold, causing glucosuria and subsequent osmotic diuresis [1]. In children, parents often notice increased daytime urination or secondary nocturnal enuresis in previously dry children. Polydipsia arises from dehydration due to osmotic diuresis, which stimulates the hypothalamic thirst center. Polyphagia reflects the energy deficit caused by impaired cellular glucose uptake; however, weight loss is common due to caloric loss in the urine, absence of insulin's anabolic effects, enhanced protein catabolism, and increased lipolysis [2].

Other frequent symptoms include fatigue and malaise. Impaired cellular glucose utilization reduces ATP production, manifesting in school-aged children as reduced concentration, irritability, and declining academic performance [1]. Hyperglycemia also negatively affects immune responses, impairing neutrophil function and predisposing individuals to infections, such as recurrent Candida infections or vulvovaginal candidiasis, which may precede diagnosis [3].

At presentation, 20%–40% of patients exhibit DKA. DKA is driven not only by insulin deficiency but also by the counterregulatory action of glucagon, cortisol, catecholamines, and growth hormone. Increased hepatic gluconeogenesis and glycogenolysis exacerbate hyperglycemia, while lipolysis produces free fatty acids that are converted to ketone bodies. Accumulation of ketones results in metabolic acidosis. Clinically, DKA presents with vomiting, abdominal pain, deep rapid breathing (Kussmaul respiration), dehydration, fruity (acetone) breath odor, and altered mental status. In young children, nonspecific clues such as irritability, failure to thrive, foul-smelling diapers, or secondary enuresis may be early indicators of DKA.

Diagnostic criteria, as defined by the American Diabetes Association (ADA) and the International Society for Pediatric and Adolescent Diabetes (ISPAD), include:

- Fasting plasma glucose ≥126 mg/dL

or

- Two-hour plasma glucose ≥200 mg/dL during an OGTT

or

- Random plasma glucose ≥200 mg/dL with classic symptoms

or

- HbA1c ≥6.5%

In symptomatic children, a single abnormal test is sufficient for diagnosis, whereas in asymptomatic cases, repeat testing is recommended to avoid misdiagnosis [1, 15].

The differential diagnosis includes type 2 diabetes, monogenic diabetes, and secondary forms. Type 2 diabetes is more likely in obese adolescents with acanthosis nigricans, hypertension, and dyslipidemia. Monogenic diabetes is suggested by negative autoantibodies, preserved C-peptide, and an autosomal dominant family history. Secondary causes include steroid therapy, cystic fibrosis–related diabetes, chronic pancreatitis, and endocrinopathies [1, 3].

In the natural history of T1DM, clinical diabetes corresponds to Stage 3b, when symptomatic hyperglycemia becomes evident. At this stage, both biochemical and clinical findings support the diagnosis [7]. Delayed recognition increases the likelihood of DKA and associated morbidity, underscoring the need for heightened

DOI: http://dx.doi.org/10.5772/intechopen.1014173

clinical suspicion in any child presenting with polyuria, polydipsia, and weight loss [2].

6. Treatment

The cornerstone of T1D treatment is lifelong insulin replacement therapy. However, successful treatment is not limited to insulin administration alone. Diabetes management should be maintained with a multidimensional approach that includes insulin therapy, medical nutrition therapy, regular physical activity, the use of diabetes technologies, education, psychosocial support, and the prevention of complications [18–20]

Insulin therapy should be initiated at the time of diagnosis in all children with T1D. The aim of treatment is to achieve normoglycemia by mimicking physiological insulin secretion and to support growth and development. Insulins are classified according to onset of action, peak time, and duration of action.

7. Insulin preparations

Insulins are classified according to their onset and duration of action (see **Table 1**):

- **Rapid–acting analogs (lispro, aspart, glulisine)**: Onset of action occurs within 5–15 minutes, with a peak effect at 1–2 hours and a total duration of action of 3–5 hours. They are administered before meals or together with meals and are effective in preventing postprandial glucose excursions.

Insulin	Brand name	Onset of action (hours)	Peak effect (hours)	Duration of action (hours)
Ultra-rapid acting	FiAsp®	0.1–0.2	1–3	3–5
Rapid-acting	Lispro (Humalog®)	0.15–0.35	1–3	3–5
	Aspart (NovoRapid®)	0.15–0.35	1–3	3–5
	Glulisine (Apidra®)	0.15–0.35	1–3	3–5
Short-acting	Regular (Humulin R®, Actrapid®)	0.5–1	2–4	5–8
Intermediate-acting	NPH (Humulin N®, Insulatard®)	2–4	4–12	12–24
Long-acting	Glargine (Lantus®)	2–4	8–12*	22–24
	Detemir (Levemir®)	1–2	4–7*	20–24
	Degludec (Tresiba®)	0.5–1.5	None	>42

Table 1.
Types of insulin and their characteristics.

- **Short-acting insulin (regular)**: Onset 30–60 minutes, peak 2–4 hours, duration 5–8 hours. Formerly standard for pre-meal use, but currently less frequently used due to its delayed onset and late hypoglycemia.

- **Intermediate-acting insulin (NPH)**: Onset 1–3 hours, peak 4–8 hours, duration 12–18 hours. Its low cost is an advantage, but it carries a higher risk of hypoglycemia.

- **Long-acting analogs (glargine, detemir)**: Provide stable basal insulin release, effective for 18–24 hours and without a peak.

- **Ultra-long–acting analog (degludec)**: Duration exceeds 42 hours. Provides a more stable glycemic profile and offers flexibility in daily injection timing.

- **Premixed insulins (lispro mix, aspart mix)**: Combinations of analog + NPH. Use in children is limited [19].

7.1 Treatment regimens

Currently, the most commonly used treatment method is multiple daily insulin injections (MDI). Approximately 40% of the daily total insulin dose is administered with long-acting analogs to meet basal needs, while 60% is provided as rapid-acting analogs at mealtimes. This method best mimics physiological insulin secretion. Continuous subcutaneous insulin infusion (CSII, insulin pump therapy) is recommended, especially in young children, in those experiencing frequent hypoglycemia, or in those unable to achieve HbA1c targets. Pump therapy allows basal rates to be adjusted according to different times of the day. Hybrid closed-loop systems integrate CGM devices with insulin pumps via algorithms. These systems perform automatic insulin adjustments, thereby keeping glucose levels within the target range for a greater proportion of time, reducing HbA1c, and lowering hypoglycemia [20].

7.2 Dose and targets

At the time of diagnosis, the insulin dose is generally 0.5–1.0 U/kg day). Insulin requirements in children with T1D vary depending on age, growth velocity, pubertal stage, residual β-cell function, dietary habits, and physical activity.

- **Infants and young children**: Insulin needs are generally lower. Insulin sensitivity is high; therefore, the daily total insulin dose is often in the range of 0.4–0.6 U/(kg day). Because feeding is frequent and irregular, preprandial bolus doses should be carefully adjusted. The risk of hypoglycemia is high in this age group, and the use of ultra-rapid analogs provides an advantage [19].

- **School-aged children**: Insulin needs are usually 0.6–1.0 U/(kg day). Ongoing growth, increased energy requirements, and physical activity necessitate careful dose adjustment. School routines and independent insulin administration skills are important [20].

- **Adolescents**: Insulin requirements increase markedly. During puberty, elevated growth hormone and sex steroids cause physiological insulin resistance. Doses may rise to 1.0–1.5 U/(kg day). The "dawn phenomenon" may increase morning insulin resistance, raising basal insulin needs. In pump therapy, basal rates may be increased in the morning hours.

After the initiation of insulin therapy, some children experience a honeymoon phase (partial remission), with reduced insulin needs and easier metabolic control. This usually occurs within weeks of diagnosis and lasts from several months up to one year, occasionally up to two years. It is due to residual β-cell function. Insulin therapy reduces glucotoxicity and lipotoxicity, relieving metabolic stress on β-cells and allowing partial recovery. This decreases exogenous insulin requirements and increases the effectiveness of endogenous insulin, [21].

Different criteria have been used to define partial remission. The most frequent include a daily insulin requirement of <0.5 U/(kg day) and HbA1c <7%. The IDAA1c (Insulin Dose Adjusted HbA1c) formula was developed for a more objective definition; values ≤ 9 indicate partial remission [22]

Although metabolic control becomes easier, insulin should not be discontinued during remission. Continuing low-dose insulin therapy may help preserve β-cell function longer and reduce the risk of DKA. This period also provides families with time to learn diabetes management and for children to adapt psychosocially. The duration of remission is influenced by age at diagnosis, sex, presence or absence of DKA at onset, residual β-cell reserve, and autoimmune burden. Older age at diagnosis, male sex, absence of DKA, greater β-cell function, and fewer positive autoantibodies are associated with longer remission. Recently, the remission phase has been considered a therapeutic window for immunomodulatory treatments. Because functional β-cells still remain, therapies such as teplizumab, abatacept, and rituximab administered during this period have been shown to better preserve C-peptide and delay progression [7]. Thus, the remission phase is regarded as one of the most critical stages in the natural course of T1DM.

7.3 Glycemic targets

The goals of glycemic management in T1DM are to support growth and development, prevent acute complications, reduce long-term risk of microvascular and macrovascular disease, and maintain quality of life. Targets should be individualized according to age, hypoglycemia risk, comorbidities, and therapeutic options. The DCCT and long-term EDIC follow-up studies demonstrated that maintaining HbA1c within the target range significantly reduces complications [23, 24].

HbA1c targets:

- <7.0% in most children and adolescents.

- <6.5% in patients with access to technologies (CGM, insulin pump, AID) and low hypoglycemia risk.

- <7.5%–8.0% in patients with a high risk of hypoglycemia, significant comorbidities, or limited access to therapy [25].

CGM-based targets:

- Time in range (TIM; 70–180 mg/dL): >70%
- Time <70 mg/dL: <4% (less than 1 hour/day)
- Time <54 mg/dL: <1%
- Time >180 mg/dL: <25%
- Time >250 mg/dL: <5% [25]

Plasma glucose targets (SMBG or CGM):

- Fasting/pre-meal: 70–144 mg/dL
- Postprandial (1–2 hours): 70–180 mg/dL
- Nighttime: >80 mg/dL (in young children, >90 mg/dL may be safer to avoid nocturnal hypoglycemia [24, 25]

7.4 Medical nutrition therapy and exercise

Medical nutrition therapy is a key component of diabetes management. Carbohydrate counting ensures appropriate adjustment of mealtime insulin doses. Healthy and balanced nutrition should be maintained, with adequate protein, fat, and fiber intake for age. Physical activity enhances insulin sensitivity but also increases the risk of hypoglycemia. Therefore, pre-exercise insulin reduction or additional carbohydrate intake is recommended [26].

7.5 Hypoglycemia and DKA management

Hypoglycemia is the most common acute complication of T1DM treatment. Symptoms occur when glucose levels fall below 70 mg/dL. Rapid-acting carbohydrate should be administered to conscious children, while glucagon is indicated in cases of severe hypoglycemia or unconsciousness [27]. DKA can occur at diagnosis or with non-adherence to insulin therapy. Management includes fluid replacement, intravenous insulin infusion, and correction of electrolyte disturbances [28].

7.6 Adjunctive therapies

Although insulin is the cornerstone of treatment, metformin may be considered for obese adolescents with insulin resistance. GLP-1 receptor agonists and SGLT2 inhibitors are under investigation, but their use in pediatric populations remains limited due to safety concerns [19].

7.7 Education and psychosocial support

Treatment success is directly related to the active participation of the child and family in diabetes management. Education programs should include insulin administration techniques, glucose monitoring, carbohydrate counting, and the management of hypoglycemia and DKA. Psychosocial support is particularly critical in adolescence to prevent treatment fatigue and adherence problems. ISPAD recommends regular psychosocial evaluation of children and adolescents.

7.8 Emerging and preventive approaches

Immunomodulatory therapies hold promise in altering the natural course of T1DM. Teplizumab, in particular, has been shown to delay progression to clinical diabetes by an average of two years in children with multiple autoantibodies and dysglycemia [7]. This finding indicates that, in the future, T1DM may not only be a treatable disease but also a preventable one.

8. Diabetes technologies (glucose monitoring and insulin delivery)

In recent years, the most significant progress in the care of T1D has been achieved in the field of diabetes technologies. These technologies not only improve glycemic control but also reduce the risk of hypoglycemia and hyperglycemia, enhance quality of life, and facilitate the active participation of families in disease management [20, 29]

8.1 Glucose monitoring technologies

- Classical method (SMBG): Finger-prick capillary blood glucose measurement has long been the mainstay of T1D management. However, due to the limited frequency of measurements, it cannot adequately capture glycemic fluctuations or reveal the risk of hypoglycemia.

- Continuous glucose monitoring: Measures interstitial glucose every one to five minutes via a subcutaneous sensor. Provides the user with real-time glucose values, trend arrows, and alarm systems. Multiple randomized controlled trials have demonstrated that CGM lowers HbA1c, increases TIR, and reduces the risk of severe hypoglycemia [30]. In addition, CGM provides reassurance to parents, especially in young children, and makes an important contribution to the prevention of nocturnal hypoglycemia. The ISPAD 2024 guidelines recommend the use of CGM in all children and adolescents with T1D [20].

- Flash glucose monitoring (FGM): Functions similarly to CGM but lacks a real-time alarm system. Glucose levels are obtained by scanning the sensor. Although FGM is less effective than CGM in lowering HbA1c, it improves hypoglycemia awareness, reduces glycemic variability, and is preferred in some countries due to its lower cost [31].

8.2 Insulin delivery technologies

- **Insulin pens:** Still the most commonly used method of insulin delivery in children. Due to the ease of dose adjustment, practicality, and portability, they are recommended as the standard form of treatment. However, the burden of multiple daily injections and injection pain may reduce treatment adherence.

- **Insulin Pumps (CSII):** Devices providing CSII. They allow variable basal rate profiles to be programmed for different times of the day and permit bolus administration with meals. Studies in children have shown that insulin pump therapy lowers HbA1c, reduces hypoglycemia, and improves quality of life [32]. ISPAD 2024 strongly recommends insulin pump therapy, particularly in young children, in patients with frequent hypoglycemia, and in those failing to achieve HbA1c targets.

- **Hybrid Closed-Loop Systems (AID):** Systems integrating insulin pumps with CGM that automatically adjust insulin dosing through algorithms. Randomized clinical trials have demonstrated significant reductions in HbA1c, improvements in TIR, and reductions in nocturnal hypoglycemia [33]. These systems have been shown to be safe and effective in children and adolescents and are increasingly becoming part of the standard of care.

Diabetes technologies are now an integral part of modern T1D management. However, access to devices, cost, national reimbursement policies, and user training remain limiting factors [34].

9. Acute complications

9.1 Hypoglycemia

Hypoglycemia is the most frequent acute complication of T1D in children and adolescents. It is characterized by plasma glucose concentrations low enough to impair brain function and may have both short- and long-term adverse consequences. To standardize clinical care and research, specific thresholds have been established. A plasma glucose level of <3.9 mmol/L (<70 mg/dL) is considered the "hypoglycemia alert level," at which treatment should be initiated to prevent progression to more severe hypoglycemia. Levels of <3.0 mmol/L (<54 mg/dL) are defined as "clinically significant hypoglycemia" and are associated with neurogenic symptoms and cognitive dysfunction. Severe hypoglycemia is characterized by profound cognitive impairment (coma or seizures) requiring third-party assistance for treatment [27].

Target glucose values have also been defined using CGM metrics. The proportion of time spent in hypoglycemia should be limited. Specifically, children with T1D should spend less than 4% of time (less than one hour per day) below 3.9 mmol/L (70 mg/dL) and less than 1% of time (less than 15 minutes per day) below 3.0 mmol/L (54 mg/dL) [25].

The clinical manifestations of hypoglycemia are grouped into three categories. Adrenergic (autonomic) symptoms include sweating, tremor, palpitations, and pallor. Neuroglycopenic symptoms comprise headache, difficulty concentrating, blurred vision, speech disturbances, confusion, seizures, and loss of consciousness. In younger children, behavioral changes such as irritability, restlessness, quietness, temper tantrums, or inconsolable crying may be the predominant manifestations [32].

Management depends on the severity of hypoglycemia. In mild-to-moderate hypoglycemia (with preserved consciousness), rapid-acting oral carbohydrate should be administered. The recommended dose is 0.3 g/kg of glucose, equivalent to approximately 9 g for a 30-kg child and 15 g for a 50-kg child. Glucose tablets or gels are preferred; fruit juice or candies may be used if glucose products are not available. Blood glucose should be re-checked after 15 minutes, and if still < 70 mg/dL, the same treatment should be repeated. Once recovery is achieved, a snack containing complex carbohydrates and protein is recommended to prevent recurrence. The treatment goal is to raise plasma glucose by approximately 3–4 mmol/L (54–72 mg/dL) [27]

In severe hypoglycemia (with impaired consciousness or seizures), urgent intervention is required. In the community setting, glucagon administration is the treatment of choice. The recommended doses are 0.5 mg intramuscularly or subcutaneously for children weighing <25 kg and 1 mg for those ≥25 kg. Novel formulations have facilitated administration, including intranasal glucagon (3 mg, ≥4 years), dasiglucagon (0.6 mg, ≥6 years), and Gvoke HypoPen (0.5–1 mg, ≥2 years). In the hospital setting, intravenous dextrose is indicated, with 2 mL/kg of 10% dextrose (maximum 0.5 g/kg) administered slowly. If necessary, a continuous infusion of 10% dextrose at 2–5 mg/kg/min may be required. Following recovery of consciousness, additional oral carbohydrate should be provided to reduce the risk of recurrence [27].

Preventive strategies are a cornerstone of management. These include regular glucose monitoring (particularly CGM use), individualized insulin dose adjustments according to meals, exercise, and illness; carbohydrate supplementation before and after exercise; routine assessment of hypoglycemia awareness; and caregiver education on the recognition and treatment of hypoglycemia, including glucagon administration. Modern technologies, such as CGM with predictive low glucose alarms and hybrid closed-loop systems, have significantly reduced both the frequency and duration of hypoglycemia in children with T1D.

9.2 Diabetic ketoacidosis

DKA is the most severe acute complication in children with T1D. At the time of diagnosis, it is observed in 20%–40% of cases. Insulin deficiency, together with elevated counter-regulatory hormones, results in enhanced hepatic gluconeogenesis, lipolysis, and ketogenesis. Clinical manifestations include polyuria, polydipsia, vomiting, abdominal pain, dehydration, Kussmaul respiration, and altered consciousness. The most serious complication is cerebral edema, which constitutes the major cause of mortality, particularly in children. Management consists of fluid replacement, intravenous insulin therapy, and correction of electrolyte disturbances, especially potassium.

9.2.1 DKA diagnosis and management

DKA is one of the most serious acute complications of T1D. Its pathophysiology involves insulin deficiency combined with an increase in counter-regulatory hormones (glucagon, cortisol, catecholamines, and growth hormone). This hormonal imbalance leads to increased hepatic gluconeogenesis and glycogenolysis, accelerated lipolysis, and excessive ketone body production. Consequently, a life-threatening clinical condition characterized by hyperglycemia, ketonemia/ketonuria, and metabolic acidosis emerges [28].

9.2.2 DKA: Definition and diagnostic criteria

According to ISPAD 2022, the diagnosis of DKA requires the presence of three fundamental criteria:

(1) **Hyperglycemia:** Plasma glucose >11 mmol/L (≈200 mg/dL).

(2) **Metabolic acidosis:** Venous pH < 7.30 or serum bicarbonate (HCO_3^-) <18 mmol/L.

(3) **Ketonemia or ketonuria:** Serum β-hydroxybutyrate ≥3 mmol/L or moderate-to-high urinary ketones.

Severity of DKA is classified according to the degree of acidosis:

- Mild: pH < 7.30 or HCO_3^- <18 mmol/L
- Moderate: pH < 7.20 or HCO_3^- <10 mmol/L
- Severe: pH < 7.10 or HCO_3^- <5 mmol/L

Clinical presentation may include polyuria, polydipsia, vomiting, abdominal pain, dehydration, Kussmaul breathing, fruity odor of the breath, and altered mental status. In children, the most serious complication is cerebral edema, which is the leading cause of mortality.

9.2.3 DKA principles of management

The main goals of DKA therapy are to correct dehydration and electrolyte disturbances, to safely resolve hyperglycemia and acidosis, to prevent complications, and to treat the underlying precipitating factor. Treatment should be conducted in specialized centers, and patients must be monitored closely with both clinical and biochemical parameters.

(1) **Fluid therapy:**

- In children with volume depletion but without shock, fluid replacement should be initiated immediately. To restore peripheral circulation, 0.9% saline is administered at a dose of 10–20 mL/kg over 20–30 minutes.
- If tissue perfusion is markedly impaired, an initial bolus of 20 mL/kg should be administered.

- The fluid deficit (5%–10%) is subsequently corrected over 24–48 hours using isotonic or half-isotonic solutions. Gradual rehydration is the goal; rapid administration increases the risk of cerebral edema and should be avoided.

(2) **Insulin therapy:**

- Intravenous insulin infusion should be commenced at least one hour after fluid therapy has been initiated.

- Regular insulin is administered as a continuous intravenous infusion at 0.05–0.1 U/(kg hour). IV bolus administration is not recommended.

- The target rate of glucose decline is 2–5 mmol/L (36–90 mg/dL) per hour.

- When plasma glucose falls to 14–17 mmol/L (250–300 mg/dL), 5% dextrose should be added to the fluids; if the decline is excessive, 10%–12.5% dextrose may be used.

(3) **Electrolyte management:**

- **Potassium:** A critical component of therapy. In cases of hypokalemia (K^+ <3.0 mmol/L), potassium replacement must precede insulin initiation. With normokalemia or mild hypokalemia, 40 mmol/L potassium should be added to IV fluids together with insulin. If hyperkalemia (K^+ >5.5 mmol/L) is present, potassium replacement should be withheld, but close monitoring is required.

- **Phosphate:** Replacement should only be considered in the presence of severe hypophosphatemia.

- **Bicarbonate:** Indicated only when pH < 6.9 and severe cardiac or respiratory dysfunction is present.

(4) **Monitoring and therapeutic targets:**

- Biochemical improvement should be gradual:

    - Glucose decline: 2–5 mmol/L per hour

    - β-hydroxybutyrate reduction: ≈ 0.5 mmol/L per hour

    - HCO_3^- increase: ≈ 3 mmol/L per hour

    - pH increase: ≈ 0.03 per hour

- Resolution of DKA is defined as pH >7.30, HCO_3^- >18 mmol/L, β-hydroxybutyrate <1 mmol/L, or normalization of the anion gap.

(5) **Prevention and management of cerebral edema:**

- The most feared complication of pediatric DKA.
- **Risk factors:** Younger age, severe acidosis, hypocapnia, rapid fluid replacement, and bicarbonate therapy.
- **Warning signs:** Headache, vomiting, altered consciousness, bradycardia, hypertension, and pupillary abnormalities.
- **Treatment:** If clinical suspicion arises, therapy should be initiated without delay. Mannitol (0.5–1 g/kg IV over 10–15 minutes) is administered; if no response is observed, a repeat dose may be given within 15–30 minutes. Alternatively, 3% NaCl at 2.5–5 mL/kg IV over 10–15 minutes can be used. Neuroimaging should not delay intervention.

(6) **Transition to subcutaneous insulin:**

- Initiated after the resolution of ketoacidosis and once oral intake is tolerated.
- The first subcutaneous insulin dose should overlap with the intravenous infusion by at least 15–30 minutes.

9.3 Hyperglycemic hyperosmolar state

HHS is rare in children but is associated with high morbidity and mortality. It is defined by:

- Plasma glucose > 600 mg/dL
- Serum osmolality > 320 mOsm/kg
- Minimal ketosis

It occurs more commonly in adolescents and often presents with clinical features resembling type 2 diabetes [28].

10. Chronic complications

Chronic complications are among the principal causes of long-term morbidity and mortality in children and adolescents with T1D; however, early detection and systematic follow-up can prevent their occurrence or slow progression. It is recommended that age-based and diabetes-duration–based systematic screening be conducted [35].

Retinopathy. Diabetic retinopathy is uncommon in childhood, but the risk increases with pubertal onset and longer diabetes duration. It is recommended to initiate a dilated fundus examination at puberty or at 11 years of age in children with two to five years of diabetes duration. After the first examination, it should be repeated every two years in low-risk patients and annually in those with risk factors, such as poor metabolic control or hypertension [35].

Nephropathy. Diabetic nephropathy is one of the major long-term microvascular complications of T1D, and although rare in childhood, early pathological changes may begin during adolescence. The earliest clinically detectable marker is increased urinary albumin excretion. Traditionally referred to as "microalbuminuria," this stage is now more appropriately described as "moderately increased albuminuria."

Screening should start at puberty or from age 11 years with two to five years of diabetes duration. The preferred method is the measurement of the albumin-to-creatinine ratio (ACR) in a first-morning urine sample. This method reduces the confounding effects of posture and physical activity, which can lead to false-positive results.

The diagnostic thresholds are as follows:

- **Normal albumin excretion:** ACR <30 mg/g creatinine (<3 mg/mmol)
- **Moderately increased albuminuria (previously microalbuminuria):** ACR 30–300 mg/g creatinine (3–30 mg/mmol)
- **Severely increased albuminuria (macroalbuminuria/proteinuria):** ACR >300 mg/g creatinine (>30 mg/mmol)

Because albuminuria can be transient, a diagnosis of persistent albuminuria requires confirmation by at least two out of three abnormal samples over a three to six month period. Conditions such as febrile illness, vigorous exercise, urinary tract infection, or poor glycemic control should be excluded as confounding factors before confirming the diagnosis.

Annual screening is recommended in eligible patients. Once persistent albuminuria is established, the first-line therapeutic intervention is the use of an angiotensin-converting enzyme inhibitor (ACE inhibitor) or angiotensin receptor blocker (ARB), even in normotensive individuals, as these agents have been shown to reduce albumin excretion and provide renal protection. Blood pressure optimization and improved metabolic control further contribute to slowing disease progression [35].

The detection of albuminuria in youth should prompt a broader assessment for cardiovascular risk factors, such as hypertension and dyslipidemia, given the strong association between nephropathy and future cardiovascular morbidity.

Neuropathy: Although typically occurring after ≥5–10 years of diabetes, an annual clinical neurological examination is recommended for all children at puberty or at 11 years of age who have had diabetes for two to five years. This examination should include sensory testing, reflexes, and assessment of autonomic function.

Dyslipidemia: As a cardiovascular risk factor detectable in early life, a fasting lipid profile should be obtained at diagnosis, particularly in children aged ≥11 years. If results are normal, repeat every three to five years. Earlier testing is appropriate with a family history of premature cardiovascular disease or dyslipidemia.

Hypertension: Because arterial hypertension accelerates microvascular and macrovascular complications, blood pressure should be measured at every visit from the time of diagnosis and interpreted using age-, sex-, and height-specific SDS values.

11. Associated autoimmune diseases in T1D

T1D is autoimmune in origin, and coexistence with other autoimmune disorders is common in children and adolescents (see **Table 2**). Autoimmune thyroid disease and celiac disease are most frequent; Addison's disease, pernicious anemia, vitiligo, and other autoimmune disorders are less common [36].

Autoimmune thyroiditis is the most prevalent comorbidity (prevalence 15%–30%). Hashimoto thyroiditis (usually hypothyroidism) predominates, while Graves' disease (hyperthyroidism) is less frequent. Hypothyroidism may impair growth, delay puberty, and worsen metabolic control. It is recommended to test TSH and thyroid autoantibodies (anti-TPO, anti-Tg) at diagnosis in all children with T1D, with repetition at least every two years if results are normal.

Condition	Screening initiation	Method	Frequency
Retinopathy	At puberty or ≥ 11 years of age with ≥ 2–5 years of diabetes duration	Fundus examination	Annually
Nephropathy	At puberty or ≥ 11 years of age with ≥ 2–5 years' diabetes duration	First morning urine albumin-to-creatinine ratio	Annually
Neuropathy	At puberty or ≥ 11 years of age with ≥ 2–5 years' diabetes duration	Clinical neurological exam (sensory testing, reflexes, autonomic assessment)	Annually
Hypertension	From diagnosis	Blood pressure measurement at every visit	Each clinic visit
Dyslipidemia	At diagnosis; if normal, repeat at 11 years, then every 3–5 years	Fasting lipid profile	Every 3–5 years (more frequently if risk factors are present)
Thyroid disease	After diagnosis, once clinically stable	TSH and anti-TPO ± anti-thyroglobulin antibodies	TSH every 2 years if antibodies are negative; annually if antibodies are positive or if a family history is present
Celiac disease	Within the first year after diagnosis, then every 2–5 years	Serum IgA and TTG-IgA (if IgA deficient: TTG-IgG and/or EMA-IgG)	Every 2–5 years; earlier if symptomatic
Other autoimmune diseases	If clinically suspected	Symptom-directed clinical assessment ± relevant autoantibodies	As clinically indicated

Table 2.
Screening for chronic complications and associated autoimmune conditions in children and adolescents with type 1 diabetes.

Celiac disease occurs in approximately 3%–8% of children with T1D. Clinical features include growth faltering, chronic abdominal pain, iron-deficiency anemia, and recurrent diarrhea; asymptomatic courses are common. The measurement of anti-tissue transglutaminase IgA (anti-tTG IgA) and total IgA at diagnosis is recommended. In cases of IgA deficiency, IgG-based assays should be used. Repeat screening if symptoms develop or if the risk remains high over time. The institution of a gluten-free diet after diagnosis benefits both growth and glycemic control.

Addison's disease: Although rare in T1D, Addison's disease (primary adrenal insufficiency) is more frequent than in the general population (<1%). Anti-21-hydroxylase antibodies indicate risk. Symptoms/signs include fatigue, hyperpigmentation, recurrent hypoglycemia, hyponatremia, and hyperkalemia. Early diagnosis is critical to prevent mortality.

Pernicious anemia: Associated with anti-parietal cell and anti-intrinsic factor antibodies; presents with megaloblastic anemia.

Vitiligo: Depigmented patches; prevalence is higher than in the general pediatric population.

Myasthenia gravis and other rare autoimmune conditions: Reported infrequently but reflect broader immune dysregulation in children with T1D.

12. Preventive strategies and emerging approaches

T1D is an autoimmune disorder that begins several years before the appearance of clinical symptoms. Consequently, the early identification of at-risk individuals is critical for the development and implementation of preventive strategies aimed at modifying the natural history of the disease.

According to the guidelines, risk is increased in children with a first-degree relative affected by T1D and in those carrying susceptible HLA alleles. Screening modalities include the measurement of islet autoantibodies (ICA, GAD, IA-2, ZnT8, and IAA), assessment of C-peptide levels, and oral OGTT. Children who test positive for multiple islet autoantibodies are considered to be at particularly high risk and may be eligible for participation in clinical trials of immunomodulatory interventions [6–7].

Recent evidence has demonstrated that immune-targeted therapies are capable of delaying progression to clinical disease. Among these, teplizumab, an anti-CD3 monoclonal antibody, is of particular importance. Teplizumab received FDA approval in 2022 for delaying the onset of clinical T1D in individuals aged eight years and older with stage 2 disease. Clinical trials have shown that teplizumab can postpone the onset of symptomatic diabetes by an average of two to three years [7]. ISPAD 2024 identifies teplizumab as the first disease-modifying therapy for T1D.

Other immunotherapeutic agents are also under investigation. Abatacept (CTLA-4-Ig) inhibits T-cell costimulation, and clinical studies have suggested that it may modestly prolong the preservation of C-peptide, although the effect appears to be limited. Rituximab, an anti-CD20 monoclonal antibody targeting B cells, has demonstrated short-term benefits in some studies, but its long-term efficacy remains uncertain. Additional investigational agents include dapagliflozin, anakinra, and low-dose anti-thymocyte globulin, all of which are currently being evaluated in clinical trials.

13. Conclusion

T1D in children and adolescents is common, complex, and lifelong. Management extends beyond insulin therapy to include glucose-monitoring technologies, insulin-delivery methods, structured follow-up, education, and psychosocial support within a comprehensive, multidisciplinary framework.

Conflict of Interest

The authors declare no conflict of interest.

Author details

Aylin Kılınç Uğurlu
Department of Pediatric Endocrinology, Gazi University Faculty of Medicine, Ankara, Turkey

*Address all correspondence to: aylin@ugurlu.org

References

[1] Classification and diagnosis of diabetes: Standards of medical care in diabetesd 2018. Diabetes Care. 2018, **41**, S13–27

[2] Shah AS, Nadeau KJ. The changing face of paediatric diabetes. Diabetologia. 2020;**63**:683–691

[3] Nathan DM; Diabetes Control and Complications Trial Research Group, SGJLPCOCMDLRCS. The effect of intensive treatment of diabetes on the development and progression of long-term complications in insulin-dependent diabetes mellitus. New England Journal of Medicine. 1993;**329**(14):977–986. DOI: 10.1056/NEJM199309303291401

[4] Lachin JM, Orchard TJ, Nathan DM. Update on cardiovascular outcomes at 30 years of the diabetes control and complications trial/epidemiology of diabetes interventions and complications study. Diabetes Care. 2014;**37**(1):39–43

[5] Yoo JH, Kim JH. Advances in Continuous Glucose Monitoring and Integrated Devices for Management of Diabetes with Insulin-Based Therapy: Improvement in Glycemic Control. Diabetes Metab J. 2023;**47**(1):27–41. DOI: 10.4093/dmj.2022.0271

[6] Herold KC, Bundy BN, Long SA, Bluestone JA, DiMeglio LA, Dufort MJ, et al. An anti-CD3 antibody, teplizumab, in relatives at risk for type 1 diabetes. New England Journal of Medicine 2019;**381**:603–613

[7] Haller MJ, Bell KJ, Besser REJ, Casteels K, Couper JJ, Craig ME, et al. ISPAD clinical practice consensus guidelines 2024: Screening, staging, and strategies to preserve beta-cell function in children and adolescents with type 1 diabetes. Hormone Research in Paediatrics. 2025;**97**:529–545

[8] Kandinov I, Knyazeva A, Lander E, Gryadunov D, Savvateeva E. Molecular Portrait of Autoantigens in Type 1 Diabetes. Biomolecules. 2025;**15**(12), 1723. DOI: 10.3390/biom15121723

[9] Dhatariya KK, Glaser NS, Codner E, Umpierrez GE. Diabetic ketoacidosis. Nature Reviews Disease Primers. 2020;**6** (40). DOI: 10.1038/s41572-020-0165-1

[10] Titmuss A, Korula S, Wicklow B, Nadeau KJ. Youth-onset type 2 diabetes: An overview of pathophysiology, prognosis, prevention and management. Current Diabetes Reports. 2024;**24**: 183–195

[11] Shah AS, et al. ISPAD Clinical Practice Consensus Guidelines 2024: Type 2 Diabetes in Children and Adolescents. Horm Res Paediatr. 2025;**97**(6):555–583. DOI: 10.1159/000543033

[12] Bhattacharya S, Fernandez CJ, Kamrul-Hasan ABM, Pappachan JM. Monogenic diabetes: An evidence-based clinical approach. World Journal of Diabetes. 2025;**16**(5):104787. DOI: 10.4239/wjd.v16.i5.104787

[13] Barbetti F, Deeb A, Suzuki S. Neonatal diabetes mellitus around the world: Update 2024. Journal of Diabetes Investigation. 2024;**15**:1711–1724

[14] Ode KL, Ballman M, Battezzati A, Brennan A, Chan CL, Hameed S, et al. ISPAD clinical practice consensus

guidelines 2022: Management of cystic fibrosis-related diabetes in children and adolescents. Pediatric Diabetes. 2022;**23**:1212–1228

[15] Libman I, Haynes A, Lyons S, Pradeep P, Rwagasor E, ling TJY, et al. ISPAD clinical practice consensus guidelines 2022: Definition, epidemiology, and classification of diabetes in children and adolescents. Pediatric Diabetes. 2022;**23**:1160–1174

[16] International Diabetes Federation (IDF). IDF Diabetes Atlas 11 th edition [Internet]. 2025. Available from: www.diabetesatlas.org [Accessed: 2025-September-29]

[17] Erlich H, Valdes AM, Noble J, Carlson JA, Varney M, Concannon P, et al. HLA DR-DQ haplotypes and genotypes and type 1 diabetes risk analysis of the type 1 diabetes genetics consortium families. Diabetes. 2008;**57**:1084–1092

[18] de Wit M, Gajewska KA, Goethals ER, McDarby V, Zhao X, Hapunda G, et al. ISPAD clinical practice consensus guidelines 2022: Psychological care of children, adolescents and young adults with diabetes. Pediatric Diabetes. 2022;**23**:1373–1389

[19] Cengiz E, Danne T, Ahmad T, Ayyavoo A, Beran D, Codner E, et al. International society for pediatric and adolescent diabetes clinical practice consensus guidelines 2024: Insulin and adjunctive treatments in children and adolescents with diabetes. Hormone Research in Paediatrics 2025;**97**:584–614

[20] Tauschman M, Cardona-Hernandez R, Desalvo DJ, Hood KK, Laptev DN, Lindholm Olinder A, et al. International society for pediatric and adolescent diabetes clinical practice consensus guidelines 2024 diabetes technologies: Glucose monitoring. Hormone Research in Paediatrics. 2025;**97**:615–635

[21] Oram RA, Jones AG, Besser RE, Knight BA, Shields BM, Brown RJ, Hattersley AT, McDonald TJ. The majority of patients with long-duration type 1 diabetes are insulin microsecretors and have functioning beta cells. Diabetologia. 2025;**57** (1):187–191. DOI: 10.1007/s00125-013-3067-x

[22] Mortensen HB, Hougaard P, Swift P, Hansen L, Holl RW, Hoey H, et al. New definition for the partial remission period in children and adolescents with type 1 diabetes. Diabetes Care 2009;**32**:1384–1390

[23] Lachin JM, Bebu I, Nathan DM. The beneficial effects of earlier versus later implementation of intensive therapy in type 1 diabetes. Diabetes Care. 2021;**44**(10):2225–2230

[24] DiMeglio LA, Acerini CL, Codner E, Craig ME, Hofer SE, Pillay K, et al. ISPAD Clinical Practice Consensus Guidelines 2018: Glycemic Control Targets and Glucose Monitoring for Children, Adolescents, and Young Adults with Diabetes, 2018. p. 105–114. DOI: 10.1111/pedi.12737

[25] De Bock M, Agwu JC, Deabreu M, Dovc K, Maahs DM, Marcovecchio ML, et al. International society for pediatric and adolescent diabetes clinical practice consensus guidelines 2024: Glycemic Targets. Hormone Research in Paediatrics. 2025;**97**:546–554

[26] Annan SF, Higgins LA, Jelleryd E, Hannon T, Rose S, Salis S, et al. ISPAD clinical practice consensus guidelines

2022: Nutritional management in children and adolescents with diabetes. Pediatric Diabetes. 2022;**23**:1297–1321

[27] Abraham MB, Karges B, Dovc K, Naranjo D, Arbelaez AM, Mbogo J, et al. ISPAD clinical practice consensus guidelines 2022: Assessment and management of hypoglycemia in children and adolescents with diabetes. Pediatric Diabetes. 2022;**23**:1322–1340

[28] Glaser N, Fritsch M, Priyambada L, Rewers A, Cherubini V, Estrada S, et al. ISPAD clinical practice consensus guidelines 2022: Diabetic ketoacidosis and hyperglycemic hyperosmolar state. Pediatric Diabetes. 2022;**23**:835–856

[29] Biester T, Berget C, Boughton C, Cudizio L, Ekhlaspour L, Hilliard ME, et al. International society for pediatric and adolescent diabetes clinical practice consensus guidelines 2024: Diabetes technologies - insulin delivery. Hormone Research in Paediatrics. 2024;**97**:636–662

[30] The Juvenile Diabetes Research Foundation Continuous Glucose Monitoring Study Group. Continuous glucose monitoring and intensive treatment of type 1 diabetes. New England Journal of Medicine. 2008;**359**(14):1464–1476

[31] Oram RA, Jones AG, Besser REJ, Knight BA, Shields BM, Brown RJ, et al. The majority of patients with long-duration type 1 diabetes are insulin microsecretors and have functioning beta cells. Diabetologia. 2014;**57**:187–191

[32] Tsalikian E, Tamborlane W, Xing D, Becker DM, Mauras N, Fiallo-Scharer R, et al. Blunted counterregulatory hormone responses to hypoglycemia in young children and adolescents with well-controlled type 1 diabetes. Diabetes Care 2009;**32**:1954–1959

[33] Jiao X, Shen Y, Chen Y. Better TIR, HbA1c, and less hypoglycemia in closed-loop insulin system in patients with type 1 diabetes: A meta-analysis. BMJ Open Diabetes Research and Care. 2022;**10**:e002633

[34] Weissberg-Benchell J, Antisdel-Lomaglio J, Seshadri R. Insulin pump therapy A meta-analysis. DIABETES CARE. 2003;**26**:1079–1087. Available from: http://diabetesjournals.org/care/article-pdf/26/4/1079/659360/dc0403001079.pdf

[35] Bjornstad P, Dart A, Donaghue KC, Dost A, Feldman EL, Tan GS, et al. ISPAD clinical practice consensus guidelines 2022: Microvascular and macrovascular complications in children and adolescents with diabetes. Pediatric Diabetes. 2022;**23**:1432–1450

[36] Fröhlich-Reiterer E, Elbarbary NS, Simmons K, Buckingham B, Humayun KN, Johannsen J, et al. ISPAD clinical practice consensus guidelines 2022: Other complications and associated conditions in children and adolescents with type 1 diabetes. Pediatric Diabetes 2022;**23**:1451–1467

Section 2

Pediatric Obesity

Chapter 2

Pediatric Obesity: A Large Problem Looming Over the Pediatric Population – an Even Bigger Problem for Adult Populations

Elizabeth E. Littlejohn

Abstract

This chapter is a first-hand account of the struggles we, as pediatric providers, are facing regarding pediatric obesity. Medical leaders are quick to urge the creation of centers to provide treatment for obesity but are reluctant to allocate the necessary funds. This problem is worldwide, worsening, and leading to unhealthy adults. How, as pediatric providers, can we ignore this ever-increasing problem? This chapter goes on to illustrate a typical case (reminiscent of adult medicine, yet increasingly common in the pediatric milieu), then reviews the diagnostic criteria and current management strategies based on the most recent 2023 American Academy of Pediatrics guidelines. Other considerations (such as the stigma of obesity and eating disorders) are discussed, and the chapter concludes by opining on future directions. Pediatric obesity is a precursor that must be addressed in the pediatric sector, where prevention is the only hope of staving off the serious ramifications of an unhealthy adult population.

Keywords: pediatric obesity, pediatric weight management, metabolic consequences of obesity, lifestyle modification, body mass index

1. Introduction

Anecdotally, I have been involved with either directing or establishing a pediatric weight management center for much of my career. After subspecialty fellowship training, I became the director of an affiliate hospital's pediatric weight management program. It was short-lived in the 1990s. After our affiliate hospital shifted to an alliance with another institution, and the weight management program was no longer part of our system of care, I set out to initiate a program at the hospital where I primarily provided patient care. The first obstacle was the lack of an ICD-9 code for pediatric obesity. The second hurdle, once there was a code, was how to pay for the components involved (nutrition and psychiatry) that could not bill insurance companies directly. I moved to a different hospital system for family reasons, where leadership desperately needed a pediatric weight

IntechOpen

management program. The pandemic (COVID-19) hit, and pediatric obesity exponentially rose. Hospital systems were hard hit financially, and the concept of adding pediatric social work or psychiatry (direly necessary for a weight management center) was put on hold. Hospital affiliations changed hands again for cost-saving and recovery post-pandemic. Now, under different leadership, all new programs are on hold while finances are reconfigured. The concern about this problem is that it affects all pediatric subspecialties, yet the key challenge lies in the hands of the primary care physician. Without a weight management program to refer to, primary care providers are left on their own or forced to refer to a subspecialist who contends with the comorbid conditions associated with obesity. In my experience, children who lose the weight also lose the comorbid conditions. Hence, the solution is to return to a normal body mass index in most cases. What we, as pediatric providers of care, must emphasize is prevention. We owe this to the children we care for and the adults they are destined to become. We need to alter this pattern now, or we risk having a very unhealthy adult population. Insurers and financial heads of institutions place too much energy on short-term gain instead of long-term health sustainability. In this chapter, I will review the current American Academy of Pediatrics (AAP) 2023 guidelines for the management of pediatric obesity (our template) and then opine on solutions for ways to implement these guidelines such that they best benefit our pediatric charges. Sitting back and watching this problem grow is not an option.

2. Case report

TC is a 17-year-old female who returned to the clinic for a follow-up visit regarding high cholesterol, nonalcoholic fatty liver disease (NAFLD), and metabolic syndrome in the setting of severe obesity. She was accompanied by her mother.

HPI: She originally came to our clinic at 13 years and 2 months of age. The parent was informed about the abnormal laboratory findings, but no recommendations were provided by her primary care provider; thus, she was referred for evaluation of the metabolic consequences of obesity. The patient has an allergy to cottonwood trees. Her mother is morbidly obese and has type 2 diabetes mellitus, hypertension, and high cholesterol. Her father is healthy. The maternal grandmother had a cerebrovascular accident, and the maternal grandfather had high cholesterol, with hypertension and type 2 diabetes mellitus. The paternal grandfather was deceased due to unknown etiology. The patient does not participate in any exercise, enjoys reading and art, and does not "like people." She is in eighth grade at a local middle school. She is currently participating in online schooling but is not performing well. She experienced menarche at 11.5 years, initially had regular menses, but then began skipping every few months. Her menses were described as starting heavy, followed by a light flow, and she experienced cramps during her periods. She reported feelings of both hot and cold, dry skin, and constant fatigue. She shares a room with her 8-year-old sister, who stays awake until 1 AM; patient herself is on the phone until 1 AM nightly. She sleeps in a bed. Her mother has polycystic ovarian syndrome. The patient denied hirsutism. She drinks milk, water, regular soda, and zero-sugar soda.

Interval since last visit 5/20/25: plan per last visit – >

- RD follow-up today to lower BMI and lipids.
- Increase fiber in diet to three tablets.
- Increase vitamin D to 50,000 IU, alternating with 100,000 IU weekly.
- Restart metformin 2000 mg daily.
- Continue Wegovy 0.5 mg weekly; escalate doses according to the schedule below.
- No levothyroxine.
- Continue CPAP.
- Check BP at Meijer and by using a home cuff; if still elevated, refer to PCP for evaluation and management.
- Continue with lifestyle modification – slowly build up the physical activity to include daily walking.
- Follow up in four months with CMP, A1C, lipid panel, vitamin D, total/free testosterone, and TFT prior.

She returned for follow-up, now a 17-year-and-4-month-old, accompanied by her mother. She takes vitamin D 50,000 IU every other week along with 100 K every other week, and 2000 mg of metformin daily since the last interval. She does not use oral contraceptives as per her gynecologist but has an intrauterine device. She takes Wegovy 1.7 mg weekly subcutaneously every four weeks, fiber tablets (three daily), and is not taking LT4 25 mg daily. She has no menses. A VP shunt was placed in February 2005, and she uses CPAP. Due to experiencing "sulfur burps," she consulted gastroenterology, which ordered an ultrasound. A registered dietitian recommended her to consume more vegetables. She was seen by a weight management clinic in a nearby city. She occasionally gets nauseous with Wegovy and takes ondansetron for the nausea. She has a therapist who provided her with a binge eating disorder book to read; she mentioned having "a little bit of a binge eating problem." She has an intrauterine device and no menses, and she noted that she needs to find a new gynecologist. Recently, she has been working on completing her General Educational Development (GED) for a high school diploma and babysitting at a daycare. She does not drive yet but plans to start driving after turning 18 years. She will soon get bifocals.

2.1 Past medical history

Past medical history: Diagnosis date: • Abnormal thyroid function test Low FT4 • Acanthosis nigricans • Acne • Chest pain in a patient younger than 17 years • Chronic hiccups 09/28/2023 • Constipation 09/28/2023 • Daily headache • Depression • Double vision • Dyslipidemia • Elevated ALT measurement • Elevated testosterone level in female • Increased free testosterone levels • Erythema of skin 07/11/2022 (Face) • Family history of Crohn's disease in her mother 09/28/2023 • Fatigue • GERD (gastroesophageal reflux disease) 09/25/2023 • High serum sodium and chloride 05/20/2025 – > dry? • Hirsutism • History of ITP at age 4; hospitalized for 7 days • History of tonsillectomy and adenoidectomy • Hyperinsulinemia • Hypotension • Increased intracranial pressure 04/10/2023 • Lightheadedness • Low serum alkaline phosphatase • Low serum creatinine • Low serum total protein level (NCS) • Metabolic acidosis • Metabolic syndrome 09/25/2023 • Morbid obesity with body mass index (BMI) greater than the 99th percentile for age in childhood 07/14/2021 • NASH (nonalcoholic steatohepatitis) 09/25/2023 • Oligomenorrhea • Orthostatic intolerance • OSA (obstructive sleep apnea) • Panic disorder (episodic paroxysmal anxiety) • Papilledema • PCOS (polycystic ovarian syndrome) • Plagiocephaly HO • Pseudotumor cerebri • Schizoaffective disorder (HCC) • Separation anxiety • Stretch marks • Total bilirubin (elevated) • Visual problems • Vitamin D deficiency

Past Surgical History: Procedure: PR Diagnostic Lumbar Spinal Puncture with Fluoroscopy or CT. Laterality: N/A - Date: 04/12/2023. Details: Lumbar puncture with opening and closure pressure performed by Martha Feher, MD, at SMH Main OR. Procedure: Tonsillectomy and adenoidectomy procedure: ventriculoperitoneal shunt. Procedure: PR Diagnostic Lumbar Spinal Puncture - Laterality: N/A Date: 04/20/2023. Details: Lumbar puncture performed by Martha Feher, MD, at SMH Main OR.

2.2 Family history

Problem Relation Age of Onset • COPD Mother • High blood pressure Mother • Diabetes Mother • Mental illness (schizoaffective, bipolar, and anxiety), migraines, fibromyalgia – Mother • Crohn's disease Mother • Irritable bowel syndrome Mother • GERD Mother • GI problem (diverticulitis) – Mother • ADHD Sister • ADHD Brother • Depression Brother • Stroke Maternal Grandmother • Diabetes Maternal Grandfather • High blood pressure Maternal Grandfather

Current Facility-Administered Medications Current Outpatient Medications Medication Sig Dispense Refill • Bupropion (WELLBUTRIN XL) 150 MG 24 hr. tablet: Take 1 tablet (150 mg total) by mouth daily. • Omeprazole (PRILOSEC) 40 mg capsule: Take 1 capsule (40 mg total) by mouth two times daily (before meals). Dispense: 60 capsules. Refill: 11. • WEGOVY 1 mg/0.5mL SC injection: Inject 0.5 mL (1 mg total) under the skin once a week. • Metformin (GLUCOPHAGE-XR) 500 mg 24 hr. tablet: Take four tablets by mouth daily (2000 mg total). Dispense: 360 tablets. Refill: 1. • Vitamin D2 (ERGOCALCIFEROL) 50,000 UNIT capsule: Take a capsule weekly, alternating with two capsules weekly. Dose on weeks 1 and 3 will be 1 capsule = 50,000 units; dose on weeks 2 and 4 will be 2 capsules = 100,000 units. Dispense: 6 capsules. Refill: 11. • Calcium Polycarbophil (FIBER) 625 mg tablets: Take four tablets (2,500 mg total) by mouth daily. • Fluticasone (FLONASE) 50 MCG/ACT nasal spray: Instill 1 spray in each nostril at bedtime. • Levothyroxine (SYNTHROID) 25 MCG tablet: Take a tablet (25 mcg total) by mouth once daily on an empty stomach. Dispense: 90 tablets. Refill: 1. • Rimegepant (NURTEC) disintegrating tablet: Take a tablet (75 mg total) by mouth as needed. • Polyethylene glycol laxative (MIRALAX) 17 GM/SCOOP powder: Take 17 g by mouth daily as needed for constipation. Dispense: 510 g. Refill: 11. • BANOPHEN 25 mg capsule: Take a capsule by mouth three times a day as needed for severe headache. Take with Compazine. • Caffeine (DIURETIC) 100 mg tablet: Take five tablets (500 mg total) by mouth daily. • Fluoxetine HCl (PROZAC) 40 mg capsule: Take a capsule (40 mg total) by mouth daily. • Levonorgestrel (MIRENA) 20 MCG/DAY IUD: 1 each (52 mg total). • Lurasidone HCl (LATUDA) 40 MG tablet: Take a tablet (40 mg total) by mouth daily.

• Prochlorperazine (COMPAZINE) 10 mg tablet • Propranolol (INDERAL) 20 mg tablet: Take two tablets by mouth 2 times a day. • Rizatriptan (MAXALT-MLT) 10 mg disintegrating tablet • Acetaminophen (TYLENOL) 500 mg tablet: Take two tablets (1,000 mg total) by mouth every 6 hours as needed. 30 tablets. • Acetazolamide (DIAMOX) 500 mg capsule: Take two capsules (1,000 mg total) by mouth. (Patient not taking: Reported on 8/28/2025.) • Betamethasone valerate (VALISONE) 0.1% cream: Apply topically. (Patient not taking: Reported on 8/28/2025.) • Mupirocin (BACTROBAN) 2% ointment: Apply topically. (Patient not taking: Reported on 8/28/2025.) • Naproxen (NAPROSYN) 500 mg tablet. (Patient not taking: Reported on 8/28/2025.) • Verapamil (CALAN) 40 mg tablet: Take a tablet (40 mg total) by mouth daily. (Patient not taking: Reported on 8/28/2025.)

Current Facility-Administered Medications Medication: ondansetron (ZOFRAN-ODT) disintegrating tablet Dose: 8 mg Route: 8 mg Oral Frequency: PRN Provider: Suad Y. A. Khalil, MD Last Rate: 8 mg Last Admin: [Information missing]

2.3 Social history on file social history

Socioeconomic History • Marital status: Single • Spouse name: None • Number of children: None • Years of education: None • Highest education level: None Occupational History • None Tobacco Use • Smoking status: Never • Passive exposure: Never • Smokeless tobacco: Never Substance and Sexual Activity • Alcohol use: None • Drug use: None • Sexual activity: None Other Topics of Concern • None Social History Narrative Lives at home with mom, younger brother, younger sister, and a cat; no father; not discussing father in Bath, MI. Grade in school: 10th. Favorite activities: Crochet, sew, and read. Immunizations are up to date (including flu shot and COVID shot).

Not currently in school, looking to go back online next year. Lives with mom, brother, sister, and a cat.

2.4 Social drivers of health plus rest of case presentation and discussion

Financial Resource Strain: Not on file Food Insecurity: Not on file Transportation Needs: Not on file Physical Activity: Not on file Stress: Not on file Intimate Partner Violence: Not on file Housing Stability: Not on file

DHx: on time; getting GED; no mention of grades.

Review of systems:

Constitutional: No fatigue, no changes in appetite, no excessive weight changes; musculoskeletal chest pain.

HEENT: No head trauma, no hearing difficulties, no nasal discharge, no sore throat.

Visual: No glasses, no blurred vision, no diplopia, no other eye problems.

Respiratory: No cough, no wheezing, no shortness of breath.

Cardiac: No chest pain, no shortness of breath, no palpitations, no syncope.

Abdominal: No abdominal pain, no bloating, no diarrhea, no constipation, no nausea, and no vomiting.

Genitourinary: No frequency, no polyuria, no nocturia/nocturnal enuresis. Irregular menses.

Neurologic: Normal coordination; no weakness, no seizures, no developmental delays.

Musculoskeletal: No joint pain, no arthritis, no fractures, no cramps.

Skin: No eczema, no rash, no itching.

Psychological: No behavior problems, no school problems, no aggressive behavior, no depression, no anxiety.

Endocrine: No cold intolerance, no heat intolerance, no polydipsia.

Objective:

Physical examination:

Vitals: BP (!) 107/59 | Pulse 88 | Ht 67.87" (172.4 cm) | Wt (!) 324 lb 1.6 oz (147 kg) | BMI 49.46 kg/m^2

Ht readings from last three encounters:

08/28/25: 67.87" (172.4 cm) (93%, Z = 1.45)*

08/11/25: 68.11" (173 cm) (94%, Z = 1.55)*

05/20/25:68.11" (173 cm) (94%, Z = 1.56)*

Growth percentiles are based on CDC (Girls, 2–20 years) data.

Wt readings from last three encounters:

08/28/25: (!) 324 lb 1.6 oz (147 kg) (>99%, Z = 2.79)*

08/11/25: (!) 322 lb 4.8 oz (146.2 kg) (>99%, Z = 2.79)*

05/20/25: (!) 326 lb 5 oz (148 kg) (>99%, Z = 2.81)*

Growth percentiles are based on CDC (Girls, 2–20 years) data.

Body mass index is 49.46 kg/m^2., 99.976%ile (Z = 3.50, 166% of 95%ile) based on CDC (Girls, 2–20 Years) BMI-for-age data available on 8/28/2025. It is 92.689%ile (Z = 1.45) based on CDC (Girls, 2–20 Years) stature-for-age data recorded on 8/28/2025. Additionally, it is >99%ile (Z = 2.79) based on CDC (Girls, 2–20 Years) weight-for-age data using information from 8/28/2025.

GENERAL APPEARANCE: Alert, cooperative, in no acute distress; general obesity; wears glasses for reading and distance.

HEAD: Mucous membranes moist; oropharynx clear.

EYES: Eyelids and eyelashes normal; conjunctivae and sclere clear; pupils equal, round, and reactive to light and accommodation.

NECK: Supple without significant adenopathy, and trachea midline; no thyromegaly present.

CHEST: Clear to auscultation bilaterally with easy respiratory effort; breast Tanner V.

HEART: Regular rate and rhythm without rubs, murmurs, or gallops.

ABDOMEN: Soft, nontender, nondistended, and no hepatosplenomegaly.

GENITOURINARY: Tanner V

MUSCULOSKELETAL: No cyanosis, clubbing, or edema is noted; no extremity musculoskeletal defects are noted.

PSYCH: Mood and affect appear normal; does not appear depressed or anxious.

SKIN: No rashes, induration, or jaundice, and no lipohypertrophy or lipoatrophy; + acne; + stretch marks; + erythematous cheeks bilaterally; + LA/lower back hirsutism; + AN.

08/04/25 10:27
Sodium: 143
Potassium: 4.5
Chloride: 107
CO2, Total: 22.0
Anion Gap: 14 (H)
Glucose: 97
BUN: 16
Creatinine: 0.69
Calcium: 9.90
Alkaline Phosphatase: 96
Albumin: 4.6
Protein, Total: 6.7
AST: 50 (H)
ALT: 82 (H)
Bilirubin, Total: 1.6 (H)
Cholesterol: 197 (H)
Triglycerides: 261 (H)
HDL Cholesterol: 35 (L)
LDL Cholesterol, Calculated: 110 (H)
Cholesterol/HDL Ratio: 5.6 (H)
25 (OH) Vitamin D Total: 61.6
Hemoglobin A1C: 5.1
Est. Average Glucose: 99.7
TSH: 3.22
Free T4: 1.42
(H): Data is abnormally high
(L): Data is abnormally low
Assessment/Plan:
In summary, TC is a 17-year-old female with:

- Obese BMI (166th% of 95th%) – > max metformin, on trial of oral GLP-1 RA, then bariatric surgery.

- Elevated free testosterone (increased bioavailable T); then within normal limits (wnl) on OCP; off OCP – elevated again; family history of hyperandrogenism (FOH); then wnl on IUD; then elevated again – continue metformin; continue with lifestyle modification (LSM) and GLP-1 RA to lower BMI and androgen levels.

- Dyslipidemia – high TC and TG, low HDL, high TC/HDL cholesterol; about the same.

- Oligomenorrhea – >Physiologic anovulation of adolescence (PAA) or other; no menses since 7/2022 – >then having menses on OCP; off OCP, having menses; then on IUD with no menses.

- HO ITP
- HO T and A
- Plagiocephaly, HO
- Elevated insulin levels; IR
- Visual problems (wears glasses for up-close and distance)
- Fatigue –> sleep hygiene issues?
- Stretch marks– >tall; UFC negative
- Acne – >androgens elevated
- Elevated ALT/AST – chronic/has had it before; follows up with GI; has had elevated ALT and TB in the past (pre-GLP-1).
- Low creatinine– >NCS
- HO VDD
- OSA – >uses CPAP
- PCOS; controlled on OCP– >FOH
- Low alk phos– >ncs
- Elevated TB >chronic/has had it before; follows with GI
- Skin erythema (cheeks bilaterally)
- Depression
- Pseudo-tumor Cerebri (HA) – just LP for Rx; now has a shunt
- Hirsutism
- Abnormal TFT –> low FT4 with normal TSH –> now TSH elevated; will trend and do Ab time 2 if rising; then wnl, again elevated with low FT4 by dialysis with normal FT4; Ab negative times two; central, subclinical, or obesity.
- HA, daily
- Metabolic acidosis
- Papilledema

DOI: http://dx.doi.org/10.5772/intechopen.1014174

- Double vision
- Increased ICP
- Panic disorder
- Schizoaffective disorder
- Separation anxiety
- Chest pain
- GERD
- Hypotension
- Light headedness
- Metabolic syndrome
- MASH
- Orthostatic intolerance
- Constipation
- FHx of Crohn's disease in mother.
- Chronic hiccups
- AN
- Low TP
- High Na Cl; dry
- High AG – >NCS
- High LDL cholesterol

PLAN:

- Continue three fiber tabs daily
- Continue* Wegovy 1.7 mg daily SQ for now; will increase at next visit if no weight loss or minimal.
- Follow up with a registered dietitian to lower lipids and BMI.

- Continue off levothyroxine for now; discontinued.
- Continue intensive lifestyle modification with daily physical activity; these habits will need to be firmly in place when/if weaned from GLP-1 RAs.
- Continue vitamin D 50,000 IU, alternating with 100,000 IU weekly; refilled. Titrate according to vitamin D level; decrease if the level continues to trend upward.
- Hold on statin; consider if LDL continues to rise.
- Continue metformin 2000 mg daily; refilled.
- FU GI, RD, HDVCH, WMC, and therapist for ongoing issues involved.
- Continue use of CPAP; repeat sleep study as indicated by sleep medicine or ENT.
- Follow up in 4 months with CMP, A1C, lipid panel, vitamin D, total/free testosterone, and TFT prior; increase Wegovy to 2.4 mg weekly if tolerating and experiencing poor weight loss.

*Weight management, chronic

Note: Use as an adjunct to diet and exercise. Escalate to the maintenance dose slowly over at least 16 weeks to minimize GI side effects.

Children ≥12 years and adolescents: Wegovy:

Initiation and titration: Initiate and adjust the dose using the following schedule. In patients who do not tolerate a dosage increase, consider delaying the increase for an additional four weeks.

Weeks 1 through 4: SUBQ: 0.25 mg once weekly.

Weeks 5 through 8: SUBQ: 0.5 mg once weekly.

Weeks 9 through 12: SUBQ: 1 mg once weekly.

Weeks 13 through 16: SUBQ: 1.7 mg once weekly.

Maintenance:

Week 17 and beyond: SUBQ: 2.4 mg once weekly (preferred); if not tolerated, it may be decreased to 1.7 mg once weekly. Note: In the STEP TEENS trial, patients continued therapy on their maximum tolerated dose.

Case discussion: This case illustrates the typical patient that we see today in our pediatric endocrinology clinics. I am a pediatrician, yet I function like an internist. If you look at all the comorbidities, they will all improve if the body mass index normalizes. The challenge is how to accomplish this task. As illustrated by this case, this patient will need bariatric surgery; however, we have a long way to go. We start with LSM, then move to medication, then surgery. If we move to surgery immediately, it could be life-threatening. Also, surgery will not be successful if LSM is not in place.

3. Diagnosis

Following comprehensive systematic reviews, the US Preventive Services Task Force issued a Grade B recommendation that pediatricians and other primary care physicians screen children and adolescents aged 6 years or older annually for obesity, defined by body mass index (BMI) percentile. Pediatricians and other primary care physicians should measure height and weight, calculate BMI, and assess BMI percentile using age and sex-specific Centers for Disease Control (CDC) growth charts or growth charts for children with severe obesity at least annually for all children aged 2–18 years to screen for overweight (BMI ≥85th percentile to <95th percentile), obesity (BMI ≥95th percentile), and severe obesity (BMI ≥120% of the 95th percentile for age and sex). In clinical practice, BMI is frequently used as both a screening and diagnostic tool for detecting excess body fat because of its ease of use and low cost. Body Mass Index is a validated proxy measure of underlying adiposity that is replicable and can track weight status in children and adolescents. Measuring BMI and assessing weight classification is a screening step that allows the pediatrician or other primary care physicians to initiate obesity evaluation. Each child with a BMI ≥85th percentile is then evaluated with a comprehensive history, physical examination, and diagnostic studies [1]. One of the difficulties in using BMI is discerning between adipose and muscle. Per the CDC, BMI is a calculated measure of a person's body weight (in kilograms) divided by the square of their height (in meters): BMI = weight (kg)/height (m).[2]. Although BMI does not directly measure body fat, it is moderately to strongly associated with other measures that capture the amount, location, and distribution of body fat. One such measure is called dual-energy X-ray absorptiometry (DEXA). It precisely measures body composition. However, DEXA scans are expensive and not widely available. Compared to direct measures of body fat, BMI is quick and simple to calculate, inexpensive, noninvasive, and easily collected during routine health care visits. Body Mass Index does not distinguish between fat, muscle, and bone mass, all of which influence a person's weight. It also does not indicate the types of adipose tissue people have or the location in the body where they carry the adipose (central, peripheral, or both).

Body Mass Index for screening is a quick, safe, and reliable measure to assess a person's weight relative to their height. They are often grouped into categories, and some BMI categories are associated with health problems. For example, a BMI in the obesity category often indicates excess weight for height. Too much weight can increase the risk of high blood pressure, high cholesterol, and other chronic conditions. Routine BMI tracking over time is useful, as it can be used to detect weight loss or weight gain and monitor the risk of health problems related to weight. For children starting at the age of 2 years, the American Academy of Pediatrics Bright Futures recommends annual BMI assessment using the CDC's growth charts. This assessment is critical for monitoring growth and development in children.

BMI is important for population health. BMI is a well-established and valuable population health measure. It has been used worldwide for decades to assess trends and make comparisons across time, geographic areas, and groups of people. BMI data help states, localities, and public health entities make decisions to improve the health of populations. For example, the CDC's Adult Obesity Maps are based on BMI data. These maps show the rate of obesity by U.S. state or territory and by race/ethnicity. The CDC also analyzes BMI data for young children enrolled in the Special Supplemental Nutrition Program for Women, Infants, and Children (WIC). This information is useful to understand how obesity numbers vary by demographic groups and track changes over time.

Body Mass Index is important for individual health. BMI is one measure that an individual and their health care provider can use to help determine chronic disease risk. For a more complete picture of an individual's health, consider BMI along with other factors, such as medical history, including existing health conditions and family history; health behaviors, such as diet, physical activity, and sleep; physical examination findings, such as blood pressure and muscle mass; and laboratory findings, such as glucose and cholesterol levels.

Body Mass Index can be assessed using BMI calculators. For adults aged 20 years and older, use the CDC's Adult BMI Calculator to calculate BMI and the corresponding BMI category. For children and teens aged 2 through 19 years, use the CDC's Child and Teen BMI Calculator. The tool calculates BMI, BMI percentile, and BMI category. In addition, the calculator plots the BMI percentile on the CDC's growth charts.

For children, obesity classifications (Class 1–3) are determined by a BMI at or above the 95th percentile and are defined by **percentiles of the 95th percentile**:

- Class 1 Obesity: At or above the 95th percentile but less than 120 percentile of the 95th percentile.

- Class 2 Obesity: At or above 120 percentile but less than 140 percentile of the 95th percentile.

- Class 3 Obesity: At or above 140 percentile of the 95th percentile.

The CDC also has computer programs for researchers and others who analyze children's growth data [2]. In an article by Etchison et al., BMI is widely accepted in determining obesity. Skinfold thickness measurements have been commonly used to determine the percentage of body fat. These authors hypothesized that because BMI does not measure fat directly but relies on body weight alone, a large percentage of athletic adolescents will be misclassified as obese by BMI. Using cross-sectional study methodology, they compared BMI and skinfold measurements as indicators for obesity in an adolescent athletic population. Anthropometric data (height, weight, percentage body fat, age, and sex) were recorded from 33,896 student-athletes (average age: 15 years; range: 11–19 years) during preparticipation physical examinations from 1985 to 2003. BMI was calculated from height and weight. The percentage of body fat was determined by measuring skinfold thickness. They found that, according to their BMI percentile, 13.31% of adolescent athletes were obese. Using the skinfold method, only 5.95% were obese. Of those classified as obese by the BMI, 62% were considered false positives by the skinfold method. In contrast, there was a 99% probability that those classified as nonobese by BMI would not be obese by the skinfold method (negative predictive value = 0.99). They concluded that BMI is a measurement of relative body weight, not body composition. Because lean muscle mass weighs far more than fat, many adolescent athletes are incorrectly classified as obese based on BMI. Skinfold testing provides a more accurate body assessment than BMI in adolescent athletes. Correct body composition data can help to provide better diet and activity guidelines and prevent the psychological problems associated with being labeled as obese [3]. Taking muscle mass into consideration is important to avoid labeling muscular athletes as obese; these are very difficult cases, as they need to be counseled on a healthful diet but not necessarily weight loss. Many of these athletes need support and reassurance that their obese BMI is acceptable if they remain physically active and muscular.

4. Treatment

4.1 Intensive lifestyle modification

Initiation of intensive lifestyle modification (LSM) is the mainstay of BMI reduction; it is required for medication and surgery to be successful. With a child, we are coping with family habits, cultural norms, and often obese parents. The growing prevalence of overweight and/or obese children is an important public health problem in both developed and developing countries. Although the association of obesity between parents and their children is well known, its underlying mechanisms are not well established. A meta-analysis by Lee et al. examined parent-child (PC) relationships in obesity and identified factors such as world region and country income level that may influence this relationship. They identified all related studies published between January 1, 2015, and May 31, 2020, by conducting a literature search using the terms "obesity," "overweight," "body mass index," "parent," "child," "associate," and "relate" in the PubMed database in English. The meta-analysis of 23 studies reporting an odds ratio (OR) for parent and child obesity associations found a significant association between parents and children who were overweight or obese (pooled OR, 1.97; 95% confidence interval, 1.85–2.10). A meta-regression analysis was then used to examine the sources of interstudy heterogeneity. The association between parent and child obesity was higher in Asia than in Europe and the Middle East, and higher in high-income countries than in middle- or low-income countries. A higher association between parent and child obesity was found when both parents were obese than when only the father or mother was obese. This study from multiple countries indicates a significant PC relationship in weight status that varies according to PC pair type, parent and child weight statuses, world region, and country income level. These results demonstrate that the risk of childhood obesity is greatly influenced by parental weight status and indicate that parents play an important role in preventing child obesity [4]. This means that altering the nutritional composition of the child requires "buy-in" by the family, including other family members like grandparents, who care for the child. Many times, one parent presents with the child, but the other parent is an "offender" or not willing to change food and activity habits. This poses a particular challenge for weight loss in the child. Or, if other caregivers or babysitters (e.g., grandparents) are not on board with LSM, this results in the child being exposed to an unhealthy environment for a significant part of the time.

5. Medication

The use of anti-obesity medications (AOMs) is new in the pediatric population. Reasons for limited use include limited data on safety and efficacy in this population, the perception that medications are not needed in this population, lack of knowledge regarding prescribing these medications, and lack of insurance carrier coverage. Three medications that are Food and Drug Administration (FDA) approved for use in children include Liraglutide (Victoza), Phentermine/Tpiramate, and Semaglutide (Wegovy) and are leading their way as tools in the arsenal toward tackling this growing problem. These approvals, along with the increasing awareness that obesity is a chronic, relapsing, biologically based medical disease and a biologically based disorder of the energy regulation system, are brandishing renewed attention to this problem [5]. Worsened by the COVID-19 pandemic [6], pediatric obesity is a growing epidemic that now requires more methods to combat this issue, and medications are increasingly used immediately with LSM. Patient characteristics that influence the use of AOMs include age, BMI and BMI trajectory, presence of obesity-related comorbidities, response to LSM, and patient/family preferences. As early as 2007, the AAP expert committee suggested the use of AOMs for children > or = to 12 years old who have a BMI ≥99th percentile or BMI ≥95th percentile with the presence of weight-related comorbidities [7]. More recently, the AAP published its Clinical Practice Guideline on the assessment and treatment of obesity [1]. These evidence-based guidelines recommend offering AOMs to children > or = to 12 years with obesity according to medication-specific indications. In all situations, AOMs should be used as an adjunct to intensive LSM. Children of 6–11 years of age who present with class 2 or 3 obesity are very unlikely to achieve durable success with LSM alone and thus should be offered therapy with AOM (off-label). In this age group, class 1 obesity with the presence of comorbid conditions such as metabolic dysfunction-associated steatotic liver disease (MASLD) or prediabetes should also prompt treatment with AOMs. Children under the age of 6 years are most responsive to LSM. Yet, patients under the age of 6 years with class 3 obesity complicated by comorbid conditions may be considered for AOM, as this represents a phenotype that is at high risk for progressive obesity, serious morbidity, and premature mortality [5]. A child <5 years of age should also have genetic testing, given the increasing pathology-specific treatments that may apply if an obesity syndrome is diagnosed (i.e., Imcivree for Prader-Willi Syndrome, clinical trial research) [8]. An exhaustive list of medications and indications for use can be found in reference [5]. In practice, we typically start with metformin, approved for use in prediabetes and type 2 diabetes mellitus in obese children, which has a modest effect on weight loss by improving insulin sensitivity and satiety, often resulting in nausea associated with eating, thus eating less than normal [9].

Another consideration is regarding the length of therapy and when to stop or what to do post-achievement of goal BMI [5]. Because AOMs work by countering the abnormal physiology, taking them away typically leads to weight gain. Treating obesity is analogous to treating any chronic condition; therefore, long-term use of medications is critical to reduce the progression and subsequent complications. This question is being studied currently by the Pediatric Endocrine Society Obesity Special Interest Group (PES Obesity SIG), which is actively monitoring children who have reached their goal BMI and the steps taken regarding AOM use (discontinuation or reduction of dose). Answers will be forthcoming, but in the interim, our experience is ongoing use of low-dose AOM while continuing intensive LSM. As we get more targeted AOMs, we will likely use a cocktail of medications to maintain goal BMI in the future.

6. Surgery

While data in the pediatric population is almost nonexistent regarding metabolic bariatric surgery (MBS), AOM use pre-surgically may be helpful in improving co-morbidities, such as diabetes, particularly in children with very high BMIs (>50 kg/m^2), to reduce the risk of surgical/anesthetic complications [5].

According to the Metabolic and Bariatric Surgery Accreditation and Quality Improvement Program (MBSAQIP), pediatric patients undergoing MBS must be managed by an accredited pediatric or adolescent medicine provider. The care team should include a licensed behavioral health specialist experienced in treating obesity, a registered dietitian, a physical therapist, and a nurse coordinator. The goals of pre-operative preparation are to diagnose and treat weight-related conditions that may affect outcomes. Patients and families must also adopt lifestyle changes that would prevent post-operative complications and maximize post-operative weight loss.

Eligibility criteria include Class 2 obesity or a BMI >120% of the 95th percentile with diagnosed comorbidities (Type 2 diabetes mellitus, hypertension, idiopathic intracranial hypertension, MASLD, slipped capital femoral epiphysis, gastroesophageal reflux disease, obstructive sleep apnea, or Blount's disease) or Class 3 severe obesity or >140% of the 95th percentile; comorbidities are not required [5]. Nutrition education, pre-operative screening labs, pre-operative weight loss goals, psychological evaluation, and physical activity goals are determined. Current or planned pregnancy, active substance abuse, medically correctable obesity, and the presence of medical or psychological issues that prevent the ability to adhere to a post-operative care plan are contraindications. The most common procedures are laparoscopic sleeve gastrectomy (LSG) and Roux-en–Y gastric bypass (RYGB). Post-operative care includes careful advancement of diet, maintaining hydration, and adequate protein intake. Supplementation with a multi-vitamin plus iron, vitamin D, calcium citrate, vitamin B12, and thiamine is required. Screening labs are monitored, and the complications are myriad (hair loss, fatigue, bruising, rashes, etc.). Dumping syndrome is common after RYGB but not LSG. The worst complication is weight regain. In the TEEN-LABS study, only 60% of adolescents maintained 20% total body weight loss following RYGB in comparison to adults. This may represent the strong genetic component of pediatric obesity or the use of weight instead of BMI in a growing population [10]. The most common post-operative complication is dehydration, which typically occurs in the first month after surgery. It is important to administer intravenous (IV) vitamins (thiamine or B1) prior to IV fluids with dextrose to prevent Wernicke's encephalopathy [10].

7. Other considerations

In the presence of obesity, disordered eating behaviors are prevalent, increasing the risk of developing eating disorders. The most frequently observed in subjects with obesity are bulimia nervosa and binge-eating disorders, both of which are characterized by abnormal eating or weight-controlling behaviors. Varied are the mechanisms underlying the interactions, including environmental and individual ones, and different approaches are needed to reduce the consequences. Evidence-based treatments for obesity and eating disorders in childhood include, as first-line approaches, weight loss with nutritional management and lifestyle modification via behavioral psychotherapy, as well as treatment of psychiatric comorbidities if not a consequence of the eating disorder. Drugs and bariatric surgery are needed in extreme cases. Future research is necessary for early detection of risk factors for prevention, more precise elucidation of the mechanisms that underpin these problems, and, in cases requiring therapeutic intervention, to provide tailored and timely treatment [11].

Children and adolescents who are overweight or obese are exposed to many forms of weight stigma, including verbal teasing by peers, social exclusion by peers, physical bullying by peers, and different expectations from adults (parents, teachers, and coaches). While other children are the main source of stigma toward obese children, teachers, coaches, parents, and healthcare providers can play a role as well. Some primary care providers do not address overweight or obese BMI during well-child checkups due to time constraints or their own discomfort with the subject. Children with excess weight suffer a great deal from weight stigma. They become more likely to have low self-esteem, depression, anxiety, and a poor body image. Studies have found that children living with obesity who face negative attitudes from peers have higher rates of suicidal thoughts and behaviors than their normal-weight counterparts. Facing weight stigma can cause health problems. These include unhealthy eating behaviors, binge eating, or trying unhealthy weight-loss options. Weight bias can also affect a child's heart health. One study found that teens who were unfairly treated due to their physical appearance had higher blood pressure, even after considering their current body weight, gender, activity level, posture, and mood. Overall, the added effects of weight bias greatly reduce a child's quality of life, from declines in physical and psychosocial health to emotional and social well-being and school functioning. All areas of a child's life are affected by weight bias [12–17].

8. Future directions and conclusion

In a recent publication in JAMA by Forrest et al., through cross-sectional analysis using mortality statistics from the US and 18 comparator high-income nations from the Organization for Economic Co-operation and Development, 5 nationally representative surveys, and electronic health records from 10 pediatric health systems, they found that the health of US children has worsened over the last 17 years. Additionally, they note that the prevalence of chronic disease in 3–17 year-olds rose, with rates of obesity along with early menstruation, sleep troubles, limitations in physical activity, depression, and loneliness all increasing from 2011–2023 [18]. Granted, the COVID-19 pandemic clearly took its toll, as it pushed an already increasing rise in diabetes even higher [18]. It unmasked other medical problems in children as well, such as obesity [6]. It is imperative now that we focus on the problem of childhood obesity to implement guidelines to curb the problem at a granular level [19], as well as at a macro-level (state and country). Research into how to best implement these guidelines [1] globally is direly needed. We must target families at all socioeconomic levels, as this problem not only imperils the underserved but the overserved as well (men more so than women [20]). Because our bodies are meant to conserve (hunter-gatherer hypothesis [21]), we must now feed ourselves judiciously; avoid the abundance of processed carbs (nutrient-poor, calorically dense, drives hunger) [22], and go back to the basics. All the treatments for obesity include the reduction of portion sizes (LSM, AOM, and MBS), focusing on the consumption of plant-based carbohydrates, lean protein, and essential fats to nourish ourselves effectively and conservatively. We must study the effects of processed carbs on the mind and body and stop succumbing to big business

DOI: http://dx.doi.org/10.5772/intechopen.1014174

pressure flooding the food market with these temptations. Already, we are seeing the effects on our children's health [23]. If we want to be the sickest nation in the world, let us keep propagating this pattern. If we want to send healthy children into the adult world, we need to act now. We are the pediatricians, and it is incumbent on us to stop this growing malady in our children.

Author details

Elizabeth E. Littlejohn
Department of Pediatrics, Michigan State University/University of Michigan Health-Sparrow, Lansing, MI, USA

*Address all correspondence to: elittlejohnmar29@gmail.com

References

[1] Hampl SE, Hassink SG, Skinner AC, Armstrong SC, Barlow SE, Bolling CF, Avila Edwards KC, Eneli I, Hamre R, Joseph MM, Lunsford D. Executive summary: Clinical practice guideline for the evaluation and treatment of children and adolescents with obesity. Pediatrics. 2023;**151**(2):e2022060641. DOI: 10.1542/peds.2022-060641

[2] BMI. About Body Mass Index (BMI), 2024. Available from: https://www.cdc.gov/bmi/about/index.html [Accessed: 2024-May-20]

[3] Etchison WC, Bloodgood EA, Minton CP, Thompson NJ, Collins MA, Hunter SC, Dai H. Body mass index and percentage of body fat as indicators for obesity in an adolescent athletic population. Sports Health: A Multidisciplinary Approach. 2011;**3**(3):249–252. DOI: 10.1177/1941738111404655

[4] Lee JS, Jin MH, Lee HJ. Global relationship between parent and child obesity: A systematic review and meta-analysis. Clinical and Experimental Pediatrics. 2022;**65**(1):35–46. DOI: 10.3345/cep.2020.01620

[5] Fox CK. Managing Pediatric Obesity Using Advanced Therapies; Practical Guide for Pediatric Health Care Providers. New york, USA: Springer; 2023. DOI: 10.1007/978-3-031-37380-0

[6] Al-Agailat L, Littlejohn E. Emerging pediatric obesity epidemic with the COVID-19 pandemic as an influence. Pediatric Annals. 2023;**52**(2):e48–e50. DOI: 10.3928/19382359-20230102-03

[7] Barlow SE. Expert Committee recommendations regarding the prevention, assessment, and treatment of child and adolescent overweight and obesity: Summary report. Pediatrics. 2007;**120**(Suppl Supplement_4):S164–92

[8] DynaMed. Obesity in children and adolescents. EBSCO Information Services. 2025. Available from: https://www.dynamed.com/condition/obesity-in-children-and-adolescents [Accessed: 2025-December-17]

[9] Vandana R, Foster CM. Metformin treatment of pediatric obesity. Pediatrics. American Academy of Pediatrics. 2021;**147**(3):e2020044982. DOI: 10.1542/peds.2020-044982

[10] Inge TH, et. al. Five-year outcomes of gastric bypass in adolescents as compared with adults. New England Journal of Medicine. 2019;**380**:2136–2145

[11] Stabouli S, Erdine S, Suurorg L, Jankauskienė A, Lurbe E. Obesity and eating disorders in children and adolescents: The bidirectional link. Nutrients. 2021;**13**(12):4321. DOI: 10.3390/nu13124321

[12] Brownell KD, Puhl RM, Schwartz MB, Rudd L. Weight Bias: Nature, Extent, and Remedies. NY: Guilford Press; 2005

[13] Eisenberg ME, Neumark-Sztainer D, Story M. Associations of weight-based teasing and emotional well-being among adolescents. Archives of Pediatrics & Adolescent Medicine. 2003;**157**:733–738

[14] Puhl R, Latner J. Obesity, Stigma, and the Health of the Nation's Children. Psychological Bulletin. Washington, D. C., USA: Americal Psychological Association; in press

[15] Puhl R, Brownell KD. Bias, discrimination, and obesity. Obesity Research. 2001;**9**:788–805

[16] Puhl R, Brownell KD. Confronting and coping with weight stigma: An investigation of overweight and obese adults. Obesity. 2006;**14**:1802–1815

[17] Storch EA, Milsom VA, DeBraganza N, Lewin AB, Geffken GR, Silverstein JH. Peer victimization, psychosocial adjustment, and physical activity in overweight and at-risk-for-overweight youth. Journal of Pediatric Psychology, Advance Access. 2006;**32**:80–89. DOI: 10.1093/jpepsy/jsj113

[18] Littlejohn E, Schein R. COVID-19 and diabetes: The tale of two pandemics. Pediatric Annals. 2024;**53**(7):e242–e243. DOI: 10.3928/19382359-20240502-01

[19] Skelly E, Littlejohn E. Implementing the American Academy of Pediatrics 2023 obesity clinical practice guidelines in a pediatric residency clinic. Medical Research Archives. 2025;**13**(9):10.18103/mra.v13i9.6783

[20] Ogden CL, Lamb MM, Carroll MD, Flegal KM. Obesity and Socioeconomic Status in Adults: United States 1988–1994 and 2005–2008. NCHS Data Brief No 50. Hyattsville, MD: National Center for Health Statistics; 2010

[21] Sharp D. The fetal matrix: Evolution, development and disease. Journal of the Royal Society of Medicine. 2005;**98**(3):130–131

[22] Good vs. Bad carbs: Benefits of minimally vs. highly processed carbs; Lauren Panoff MPH. medically reviewed by Aviv Joshua, MS, RDN, 2025. Available from: https://www.verywellhealth.com/good-vs-bad-carbs-8778009 [Accessed: 2026-November-01]

[23] Forrest CB, et. al. Trends in US children's mortality, chronic conditions, obesity, functional status, and symptoms. JAMA. 2025;**334**(6): 509–516. DOI: 10.1001/jama.2025.9877

Chapter 3

The Role of Endocrine Factors in Childhood Obesity

Harrison Samuel and Helen Harrison

Abstract

Paediatric obesity is a growing global health challenge and a recurring theme across this book, because it sits at the intersection of endocrine dysfunction, clinical practice, and public health. This chapter examines how excess adipose tissue acts as an active endocrine organ, disturbing appetite control, linear growth, and metabolic homeostasis. It brings together evidence on insulin resistance, leptin resistance, ghrelin dysregulation, and altered adipokine signalling, showing how these changes both follow and drive persistent adiposity, metabolic syndrome, type 2 diabetes risk, and fatty liver disease. The chapter also distinguishes common multifactorial obesity from less frequent but clinically important endocrine and genetic disorders, including hypothyroidism, Cushing's syndrome, hypothalamic obesity, growth hormone dysregulation, and monogenic defects of the leptin–melanocortin pathway. Using a phenotype-based framework, it outlines the red flags that should prompt targeted biochemical or genetic investigation rather than routine testing. Management is presented as a continuum of care. Family-centred lifestyle modification remains first-line, while glucagon-like peptide-1 receptor agonists, bariatric surgery, and targeted therapies such as setmelanotide may have a role in selected patients. The chapter closes by emphasising shared decision-making, culturally appropriate counselling, nursing-led screening and education, family physician coordination, and the need to link clinic-based care with school, food-environment, and community interventions, especially in resource-limited settings.In doing so, the chapter contributes a practical, evidence-informed guide that bridges endocrine science with day-to-day family medicine, while giving the wider volume a clear focus on prevention, early detection, and equitable long-term care for children and families.

Keywords: paediatric obesity, endocrine disruption, leptin resistance, insulin resistance, ghrelin dysregulation, nurse screening, family physician management

1. Introduction

1.1 Overview

Childhood obesity, the abnormal or excessive accumulation of adipose tissue that impairs health, has shifted from a problem largely confined to wealthy nations to a global public-health emergency affecting children in every region of the world.

IntechOpen

Rates of overweight and obesity in children and adolescents have risen sharply over recent decades, with a growing share of cases now occurring in low- and middle-income countries (LMICs) [1]. This trend has immediate clinical implications for growth, psychosocial well-being, and cardiometabolic risk in childhood, as well as profound long-term consequences, since excess weight in childhood frequently persists into adult life [2, 3].

1.2 Why does an endocrine perspective matter?

Explaining paediatric obesity solely as an outcome of dietary choice or physical inactivity is incomplete. Adipose tissue itself acts as an active endocrine organ, secreting adipokines and cytokines that communicate with the central nervous system, liver, muscle, and pancreas to regulate appetite, substrate use, and systemic inflammation. The endocrine disturbances associated with excess adiposity, notably insulin resistance, altered adipokine signalling and dysregulated appetite hormones, not only result from weight gain but also feedback to promote further energy storage, creating metabolic dysfunction [4].

1.3 Key hormonal pathways implicated in paediatric obesity

Several hormone systems play central roles in the onset and maintenance of excess weight in children:

- Insulin and insulin resistance: Hyperinsulinaemia and reduced insulin sensitivity commonly develop with excess fat and are pivotal in the emergence of dysglycaemia and fatty liver in youth [3, 5].

- Leptin and central appetite control: Leptin levels increase with fat mass, but central leptin resistance blunts satiety signalling; the resulting mismatch.

- Contributes to continued excess intake and impaired energy regulation [4].

- Ghrelin and gut peptides: Changes in orexigenic and anorexigenic gut hormones alter hunger and reward pathways and interact with adipose-derived signals to shape eating behaviour.

- Adipokines and chronic low-grade inflammation: Imbalanced secretion of adiponectin, resistin, and pro-inflammatory cytokines creates a chronic inflammatory state that promotes insulin resistance and early vascular risk [4].

Understanding which pathways predominate in an individual child informs assessment, monitoring, and more targeted interventions.

1.4 Endocrine pathophysiology and environmental modifiers

Early-life nutrition, sleep patterns, psychosocial stress, and exposure to endocrine-disrupting chemicals (EDCs) alter metabolic programming and modify the endocrine response to obesity [6, 7]. Epidemiological and mechanistic studies increasingly implicate perinatal exposures and certain environmental pollutants in heightened obesity risk and altered hormone action, offering explanations for rapid population shifts that cannot be accounted for by genetics alone.

1.5 When does obesity signal a primary endocrine disorder?

Although most paediatric obesity is multifactorial, a small but clinically important subset of children has obesity driven predominantly by primary endocrine or monogenic disorders (for example, Cushing syndrome, untreated hypothyroidism, hypothalamic injury, or rare monogenic defects in the leptin–melanocortin pathway) [8, 9]. Early-onset severe obesity, stunted linear growth, developmental delay, or unusual fat distribution are 'red flags' that should prompt specific endocrine investigation rather than routine lifestyle counselling [8].

This chapter offers a thorough review of the endocrine factors contributing to childhood obesity. It begins by discussing the current global epidemiology, highlighting the rising prevalence in LMICs. It then examines the complex biological connections between obesity and metabolic syndrome, with a particular focus on the role of key hormones. A framework for the clinical evaluation and differential diagnosis of rare endocrine causes is presented, followed by a synthesis of evidence-based management and prevention strategies, with a particular emphasis on the critical roles of nurses and family physicians in an integrated, multidisciplinary approach.

2. Definition and global epidemiology of childhood obesity

2.1 Definition

The clinical definition of childhood obesity is a crucial first step in its assessment and management. Unlike in adults, where a single body mass index (BMI) cut-off is used, the diagnosis in children must account for the continuous physiological changes that occur during growth and puberty. For children and adolescents aged 5–19 years, the World Health Organization (WHO) defines overweight as BMI-for-age >1 standard deviation (SD) and obesity as BMI-for-age >2 SD above the WHO Growth Reference median; for children under 5 years, weight-for-height >3 SD defines obesity [3]. These age and sex-specific percentile charts are the accepted gold standard for paediatric providers to track growth and identify when intervention is needed [3].

2.2 Global prevalence and trends in childhood obesity

The prevalence of overweight and obesity among children and adolescents has risen dramatically in recent decades. Global estimates indicate a large and growing burden of excess weight in youth, with multiple recent syntheses and population-level studies documenting steep increases over the past three decades [1, 2]. Over 390 million children and adolescents aged 5–19 years were overweight in 2022. The prevalence of overweight (including obesity) among children and adolescents aged 5–19 has risen dramatically from just 8% in 1990 to 20% in 2022. The rise has occurred similarly among both boys and girls: in 2022, 19% of girls and 21% of boys were overweight [1]. These increases represent roughly a 1.5–2-fold rise over the past two decades, reflecting a genuine and sustained global trend [1, 2].

2.3 Regional patterns

The rise in childhood overweight and obesity has been heterogeneous across regions. The highest current prevalence is reported in parts of the Middle East and certain Pacific Island states. At the same time, the fastest recent increases have occurred in East and Southeast Asia and parts of Latin America [1, 2]. Once seen mainly in high-income countries, excess weight is now widespread across all world regions and socioeconomic strata [2]. Several modelling studies warn that, if current trends continue, prevalence will keep climbing through mid-century, with significant regional variation in timing and magnitude [2, 10].

2.4 Trends in LMICs

There is clear and growing evidence that LMICs are undergoing rapid increases in childhood overweight and obesity. Although many low-resource countries still have lower absolute prevalence than high-income nations, the pace of rise is rapid as diets, physical activity, and urban lifestyles change [2]. For example, WHO analyses estimate that nearly half of overweight children under age five now reside in Asia, and the number of overweight young children in Africa has risen substantially since 2000 [4]. These shifting burdens underscore the urgent need for targeted prevention strategies in LMICs, where health system capacity is often limited and access to specialist services remains constrained [4].

3. Pathophysiology of endocrine imbalance in childhood obesity

Energy homeostasis is tightly regulated by the central nervous system, which continuously integrates hormonal signals from the gastrointestinal tract, pancreas, and adipose tissue. In paediatric obesity, this finely tuned network becomes disrupted: altered gut-brain signalling [8, 11], insulin and leptin resistance [9, 12–16], and adipose-derived inflammatory mediators [4, 11–14] produce an endocrine milieu that both initiates and sustains excess weight gain and metabolic dysfunction.

Chronic excess adiposity triggers adaptive responses in multiple hormonal axes (e.g., insulin, leptin, ghrelin, adipokines, thyroid hormone) [11, 12]. Elevated adipokines and inflammatory cytokines from enlarged fat depots promote insulin resistance, while elevated leptin levels are countered by central resistance. Gut hormone responses (ghrelin, GLP-1, etc.) are blunted, reinforcing overeating [8, 17]. Adipose tissue is now recognised as an active endocrine organ that secretes many adipokines and cytokines. With excess visceral fat, the adipokine profile shifts towards pro-inflammatory and diabetogenic patterns (reduced adiponectin; increased TNF-α, IL-6, resistin), which underlie insulin resistance and early vascular risk in children [4, 13, 14]. This chronic low-grade inflammatory state – metaflammation – arises from the inflamed adipose depot and drives systemic metabolic dysfunction [4, 12, 14].

Recent reviews summarise these adipokine changes and their downstream cardiometabolic implications in youth.

3.1 The hormonal–metabolic nexus: Adipose tissue as an endocrine organ

For clarity, key hormones in childhood obesity are summarised in **Table 1**. Excess visceral fat increases the secretion of leptin and inflammatory adipokines while reducing insulin-sensitising adiponectin [4, 13]. These changes impair insulin and leptin signalling and promote hepatic steatosis and dyslipidaemia [14, 17]. Affected adipose and liver tissue release free fatty acids and cytokines that further impair insulin signalling in muscle and other organs. **Table 1**

Hormone system	Function in the healthy state	Dysregulated function in paediatric obesity	Clinical consequences
Leptin	Adipocyte-derived signal of long-term energy stores suppresses appetite via hypothalamic pathways	Hyperleptinaemia with central (hypothalamic) leptin resistance – impaired transport/signalling across the blood–brain barrier and intracellular blockade	Persistent hyperphagia, impaired satiety, and difficulty achieving sustained weight loss contribute to altered pubertal timing and metabolic inflammation [14]
Ghrelin	Stomach-derived orexigenic peptide rises pre-prandially and falls after meals to stimulate or terminate feeding	Blunted post-prandial suppression and altered pre/post-meal dynamics	Continued hunger after meals, increased meal size/frequency, and difficulty with satiation [7, 16]
Insulin	Facilitates glucose uptake and storage in muscle, liver, and adipose tissue; signals satiety centrally	Peripheral insulin resistance with compensatory hyperinsulinaemia; impaired central insulin satiety signalling	Prediabetes and type 2 diabetes risk, dyslipidemia, hypertension, non-alcoholic fatty liver disease (NAFLD)/MAFLD [8, 11]
Adiponectin	Adipokine that enhances insulin sensitivity and has anti-inflammatory effects	Paradoxical reduction in circulating adiponectin, despite increased fat mass	Worsening insulin resistance, promotion of chronic low-grade inflammation ('metaflammation'), and increased cardiometabolic risk [4, 13]
Growth hormone (GH)	Promotes linear growth, lipolysis, and preservation of lean mass	Relative suppression of GH secretion in obesity (functional, reversible)	Increased fat mass and reduced lean mass may influence final height if true GHD (differentiate functional suppression from true deficiency) [18]
Cortisol/HPA axis	Regulates glucose metabolism and stress responses; episodic increases mobilize energy	Relative activation of the HPA axis and, in pathological states, sustained glucocorticoid excess (Cushing's)	Central adiposity, impaired linear growth (in children with Cushing's), hypertension, insulin resistance, and increased cardiometabolic risk [13, 19]

Table 1.
Key endocrine–metabolic disturbances in childhood obesity: Summary of normal function, obesity-related dysregulation, and principal clinical consequences.

highlights the major hormones involved, their normal functions, and how they are altered in paediatric obesity.

3.2 Leptin and the pathophysiology of leptin resistance

Leptin, produced proportionally to fat mass, normally signals satiety to hypothalamic circuits. In common paediatric obesity, leptin concentrations are elevated, but the brain becomes resistant to its satiety signal. Mechanisms implicated include impaired leptin transport across the blood–brain barrier and inflammatory-mediated intracellular blockade of leptin receptor signalling (notably SOCS proteins) [13, 15]. Work over the last five years has further highlighted hypothalamic nutrient-sensing pathways, including mTOR signalling in proopiomelanocortin (POMC) neurons, as important contributors to leptin resistance, linking cellular nutrient sensing to impaired appetite regulation [15]. These mechanistic advances help explain why behavioural measures alone often fail to produce sustained satiety and weight loss in affected children.

3.3 Ghrelin and the dysregulation of appetite

Ghrelin, an orexigenic stomach hormone, normally rises pre-meal and falls after eating. In many children with obesity, the expected post-prandial suppression of ghrelin is blunted – a pattern that permits continued hunger after meals and compounds leptin resistance to produce a strong biological drive to overeat [8, 17]. Recent paediatric and translational studies confirm persistent abnormalities in gut–brain appetite signalling in obese youth and point to these pathways as therapeutic targets for newer agents that mimic or potentiate satiety.

hormones [20].

3.4 Insulin resistance and the development of metabolic syndrome

Insulin resistance is central to the metabolic consequences of paediatric obesity: peripheral tissues become less responsive to insulin, and the pancreas contributes to dysglycaemia, dyslipidaemia, and fatty liver (metabolic-associated fatty liver disease [MAFLD]) in susceptible children [12–14, 17]. Mechanisms include adipose-derived free fatty acids and inflammatory mediators that impair insulin signalling, progressive β-cell stress, and ectopic lipid deposition in the liver and muscle. Clinical and mechanistic reviews highlight the prominence of MAFLD and cardiometabolic risk in severely obese youth, reinforcing the need for early identification and management of insulin resistance in paediatric practice [17].

4. Rare endocrine and genetic causes of childhood obesity

Although most childhood obesity is multifactorial and lifestyle-related, a small but important minority of children have obesity as a primary manifestation of an endocrine or genetic disorder. These cases require a different diagnostic pathway and, in some instances, allow for specific targeted therapies. In routine practice, endocrinopathies and monogenic causes account for well under 1% of presentations,

Clinical 'red flag'	Suspected primary disorder(s)	Appropriate next steps
Very early-onset obesity (< four years of age)	Monogenic defects (e.g., MC4R, LEP, LEPR), syndromic obesity	Consider genetic testing, guided by phenotype and family history. [20, 22]
Rapid weight gain with faltering linear growth	Hypothyroidism, Cushing's syndrome, Growth Hormone deficiency	Targeted biochemical tests (e.g., TSH, free T4, IGF-1) [18, 22]
Extreme, pathological hyperphagia	Monogenic defects (e.g., MC4R, POMC defects), Prader–Willi syndrome, hypothalamic injury	Consider genetic testing, especially for leptin–melanocortin pathway genes [20, 24]
Syndromic features (developmental delay, dysmorphism, organ anomalies)	Prader–Willi syndrome, Bardet–Biedl syndrome, Alström syndrome	Referral to a medical geneticist, multidisciplinary team evaluation [20, 21]
Unusual fat distribution (central with limb-sparing)	Cushing's syndrome, Hypothalamic obesity	Prompt biochemical testing (e.g., salivary cortisol) [19, 22]
Hypogonadism (in males)	Hypogonadism, Hypothalamic injury	Endocrine evaluation and appropriate hormone testing. [19, 22]

Table 2.
Clinical 'red flags' for investigating rare causes of obesity.

but clinicians must recognise the clinical patterns that should trigger focused evaluations [16, 21].

4.1 How to recognise a suspect case: Clinical 'red flags'?

Patterns that should prompt further investigation include early onset (infancy or < three years), rapid weight gain with faltering linear growth (short and fat), pathological hyperphagia (insatiable food-seeking), syndromic features (developmental delay, dysmorphism, retinal/renal anomalies), or clinical stigmata of endocrine disease (goitre, Cushingoid features, marked growth failure) [16]. Clinical guidelines advise a phenotype-driven approach: targeted biochemical testing and genetic referral when red flags are present, rather than routine screening of all children with common obesity [16, 22]. For a concise clinical checklist of red flags and suggested next steps, see **Table 2**.

4.2 Monogenic (non-syndromic) obesity

Single-gene defects that disrupt the leptin–melanocortin pathway cause severe early-onset obesity with hyperphagia. Heterozygous melanocortin 4 receptor (MC4R) variants are the most common monogenic causes are identified in variable proportions of severely obese cohorts; rarer biallelic defects (e.g., LEP, LEPR, POMC, PCSK1) produce more severe phenotypes [16, 21]. Genetic testing is indicated when the clinical phenotype fits, as a molecular diagnosis alters management, genetic counselling and access to precision therapies (for selected defects) [16, 20].

4.3 Syndromic genetic obesity

Syndromic forms (e.g., Prader–Willi, Bardet–Biedl, Alström) present with obesity alongside developmental, sensory, or organ-system abnormalities.

Prader–Willi syndrome – characterized by infantile hypotonia, later hyperphagia, and high ghrelin – remains the exemplar; recognition of extrasomatic clues directs genetic referral and multidisciplinary care [16, 20].

4.4 Classical endocrine disorders that cause weight gain

Certain endocrine conditions classically present with weight gain in children; prompt recognition is important because targeted treatment often restores metabolic balance and permits catch-up growth [16, 23].

4.4.1 Hypothyroidism

Hypothyroidism typically manifests with unexplained weight gain accompanied by slowed linear growth and lethargy. The diagnosis is biochemical, with an elevated thyroid-stimulating hormone and low free thyroxine, and levothyroxine replacement usually normalises the metabolic rate and permits growth recovery [18, 23].

4.4.2 Cushing's syndrome

Chronic glucocorticoid excess produces central (truncal) adiposity, poor linear growth, and the characteristic stigmata of cortisol excess. Diagnosis depends on biochemical confirmation (for example, 24-hour urinary free cortisol, late-night salivary cortisol and dexamethasone suppression testing, along with imaging, are used to localize the source; management is directed at the underlying cause (surgical removal where appropriate or medical inhibition of steroidogenesis [16, 23].

4.4.3 Growth hormone deficiency

Presents with short stature accompanied by increased fat mass and characteristic body composition changes. Biochemical evaluation reveals low insulin-like growth factor-1 (IGF-1) levels and inadequate responses to standardised GH stimulation tests. Treatment with recombinant human growth hormone restores linear growth velocity and reduces adiposity, resulting in significant improvements in body composition [19].

4.4.4 Hypothalamic obesity

Damage to ventromedial hypothalamic centres most commonly occurring after craniopharyngioma resection, traumatic injury, or other hypothalamic insults – results in profound, frequently treatment-resistant weight gain driven by marked hyperphagia and a fall in resting energy expenditure. Management is multidisciplinary and focused on caloric control, behavioural strategies, and endocrine replacement, where needed; emerging pharmacotherapies (notably GLP-1 receptor agonists) have shown promise in selected patients but require specialist oversight [23–25].

4.4.5 Insulinoma (rare)

A child with an insulin-secreting tumour may present with episodes of hypoglycaemia, which trigger compensatory overeating and weight gain. Diagnosis is established by demonstrating inappropriately high insulin levels during hypoglycaemia, and surgical resection is usually curative [21].

4.5 Diagnostic strategy and the role of genetic testing

A staged, phenotype-driven strategy is most efficient: careful growth plotting and focused clinical assessment → targeted biochemical tests when red flags are present (e.g., TSH, cortisol, IGF-1) → consider gene panels for early-onset severe obesity or syndromic presentations [9]. Broad, indiscriminate endocrine panels in otherwise typical obesity are low-yield; targeted testing increases diagnostic yield and informs therapy and counselling.

4.6 Treatment implications – targeted therapies and multidisciplinary care

A molecular or endocrine diagnosis can open targeted therapeutic options.

Setmelanotide (an MC4R agonist) has demonstrated clinically meaningful reductions in hunger and weight in individuals with specific genetic defects (POMC, LEPR).

PCSK1, and some syndromic forms; robust trials and regulatory approvals over the last five years have made precision therapy a reality for some patients [10, 26]. For other conditions (hypothyroidism, Cushing's, GH deficiency), disease-specific endocrine therapy or surgery remains the effective intervention. Regardless of the cause, management is best delivered by a multidisciplinary team that includes endocrinologists, geneticists, dietitians, psychologists, and primary care providers, with long-term follow-up [16, 20].

5. Clinical evaluation and screening

Timely detection and organised screening programs are essential prerequisites for the successful prevention and treatment of paediatric obesity. Nurses and family physicians provide complementary roles. Nurses commonly perform routine height and weight checks in clinics, schools, and community programmes. Family physicians review those data, assess for related health problems, decide what investigations are needed, and arrange referrals when appropriate. Regular measurement and plotting of BMI over time allow detection of rising trends before complications develop. Repeated assessment at routine well-child visits gives clinicians multiple opportunities to notice a sustained upward trend in BMI percentile and to act early [6]. Primary care teams may consult **Table 2** when determining which children need targeted endocrine or genetic evaluation.

5.1 The nurse's role: Screening, education, and referral

Nurses are often the first to identify children at risk. Their tasks include accurate measurement of height and weight, calculation of BMI-for-age, and plotting results on standard growth charts, such as the WHO or Centers for Disease Control and Prevention (CDC) charts. Nurses also have an important educational role. They give parents practical advice on feeding, physical activity, sleep, and limits on screen time, and they help families understand what the growth charts mean. When nurses observe rapid weight gain, unusual growth patterns, signs that suggest an endocrine problem, or troubling behaviours such as extreme food-seeking, they should prompt a clinical review by a physician [27].

Programs led by school or community nurses that combine family-centred education with practical support have shown measurable improvements in children's diet and activity [27, 28].

5.2 The family physician's role: Diagnosis, comorbidity screening, and referral

The family physician or paediatrician builds on screening findings and performs a focused assessment. This includes reviewing growth velocity and BMI trends, taking a history of diet, activity, sleep, and family illness, and examining for complications such as high blood pressure, skin changes consistent with insulin resistance, or hepatomegaly [29]. Guidelines recommend targeted laboratory screening for cardiometabolic risk according to the child's age and risk profile. Common tests for older children or those with additional risk include fasting glucose, glycated haemoglobin (HbA1c), and a lipid profile. Detecting acanthosis nigricans should prompt assessment for insulin resistance. When signs point to a possible endocrine cause, the physician orders targeted tests such as thyroid function or IGF-1 and refers the child to paediatric endocrinology.

5.3 Practical screening actions

At each well-child visit:

- Measure height and weight, calculate BMI, and plot it on the appropriate chart. A BMI ≥ 95th percentile indicates obesity, while a BMI in the 85–95th percentile range indicates overweight. Assess growth velocity and note if percentiles are crossed rapidly. [3, 6, 9]

- Record age-appropriate blood pressure, inspect the skin for acanthosis nigricans, and palpate for hepatomegaly.

- Order biochemical tests guided by age and clinical profile; commonly, this includes fasting glucose or HbA1c and a lipid profile. **Figure 1** shows the structured pathway for screening and assessment of paediatric obesity in primary care.

5.4 Screening in resource-limited settings

In LMICs, simple, low-cost methods are essential. Accurate height and weight measurement and plotting remain the core of screening. When laboratory services are scarce, clinicians use growth patterns, blood pressure, and skin signs to decide who needs closer follow-up or specialist referral. Regular nurse-led screening, training in respectful communication, and community prevention activities are practical and affordable priorities. Routine endocrine or genetic testing without red flags should be avoided; resources must focus where the yield will be highest [23].

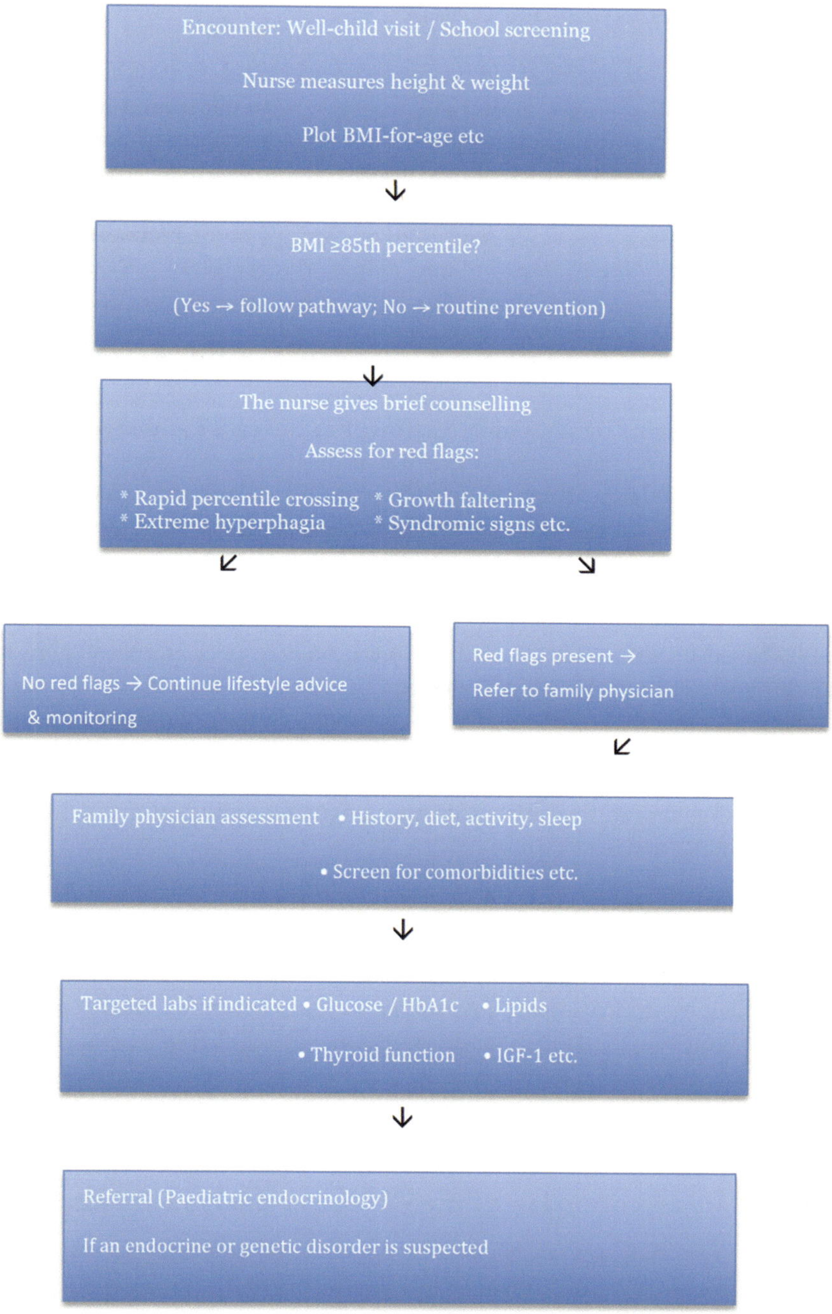

Figure 1.
Screening pathway for childhood obesity in nurses and family physicians (author-generated). Source: Based on practice guidelines and screening literature [6, 16, 23, 25].

5.5 Multidisciplinary care and next steps

A finding of excess weight should prompt a coordinated, family-centred care plan focused on achievable changes in diet and activity, with continued follow-up in primary care [6]. Referral to dietitians, exercise programmes and behavioural support should be made when available. Nurses and family physicians remain central to monitoring progress, improvements such as staff training in measurement techniques, brief counselling skills, and routine clinic systems increase the likelihood that at-risk children will be identified and managed effectively [28–30].

6. Management strategies: Endocrine-targeted and lifestyle approaches

Effective care begins by matching treatment to the cause and severity. For most children, the main drivers are environmental and behavioural; for these, structured, family-centred lifestyle treatment is first-line [6, 29]. A minority have a specific endocrine or genetic cause, requiring targeted therapy [16].

6.1 Family-based lifestyle treatment as first-line

Family-based programmes combining nutritional advice, increased activity, and behavioural support are the cornerstone of management. Interventions that involve parents, set measurable goals, and provide regular follow-up produce the most consistent improvements in weight and metabolic outcomes [28]. Practical advice includes eliminating sugar-sweetened drinks, increasing fruit and vegetable intake, promoting shared healthy mealtimes, ensuring daily activity, adequate sleep, and reducing sedentary time.

6.2 When to add medication?

Pharmacotherapy is an option when structured programmes do not achieve benefits or when complications require early weight reduction. Current evidence supports glucagon-like peptide-1 receptor agonists (GLP-1 RAs):

- Liraglutide has shown benefits in children as young as six years old in recent randomised controlled trials [31, 32].

- Semaglutide has produced significant BMI reductions in adolescents in the STEP TEENS trial [24].

Metformin is often used in adolescents with insulin resistance or impaired glucose tolerance; it improves metabolic markers, though its effect on weight is modest. Clinical decisions require careful family discussion and, where possible, paediatric endocrinology input.

6.3 Treatments directed at specific endocrine or genetic causes

Targeted therapy changes outcomes when specific causes are found:

- Hypothyroidism: Levothyroxine restores growth and metabolism [19].
- Cushing's syndrome: Requires surgical or medical therapy to correct cortisol excess [16].
- Monogenic leptin–melanocortin defects: Setmelanotide, an MC4R agonist, reduces hunger and weight in children with specific mutations [10, 26].
- Lipodystrophy: Metreleptin improves metabolic complications [33].
- Polycystic ovary syndrome (PCOS) in adolescents: Managed with lifestyle measures, metformin, and hormonal therapy [25].

6.4 Role of bariatric surgery

Metabolic and bariatric surgery is reserved for adolescents with severe, treatment-resistant obesity and major comorbidities. Surgery produces durable weight loss and cardiometabolic improvement but requires a multidisciplinary assessment and lifelong follow-up. Updated American Society for Metabolic and Bariatric Surgery (ASMBS)/International Federation for the Surgery of Obesity and Metabolic Disorders (IFSO) guidelines outline referral criteria and emphasise limiting surgery to specialised centres [34].

6.5 Practical principles for clinical decision-making

Management should consider age, severity, comorbidities, and red flags. Begin with lifestyle care, escalate to pharmacotherapy for persistent severe obesity, and pursue endocrine/genetic evaluation when indicated. Shared decision-making with families, clear communication about realistic goals, and long-term support are essential [6, 25].

6.6 Health systems and prevention

Clinical care must be integrated with prevention strategies. School and community programmes, healthier food environments, and public policies to reduce obesogenic exposures reinforce clinical efforts. In resource-constrained settings, nurse-led screening and culturally adapted family interventions remain the most practical priorities [27–29].

7. Conclusion

Childhood obesity is a chronic endocrine-metabolic condition with lifelong consequences. Most cases result from environmental and behavioural influences interacting with genetic susceptibility, producing secondary hormonal disturbances such as leptin resistance, hyperinsulinaemia, and impaired ghrelin suppression [4]. A minority present with primary endocrine or genetic disorders such as hypothyroidism, Cushing's syndrome, or MC4R pathway defects, where targeted therapy can transform outcomes [10, 16, 18, 26]. Long- term strategy

[6, 16]. Advances in therapy now include GLP-1 receptor agonists, effective from middle childhood, and bariatric surgery for selected adolescents, both of which achieve significant weight reduction and comorbidity improvement [24, 26, 31–34]. Addressing the epidemic requires clinical and public-health synergy. Policies promoting healthier school environments, reducing sugary drink access, and supporting community activity are essential to prevention [1, 25]. In LMICs, empowering nurses and family physicians to screen and counsel families early is crucial [25, 29]. With continued research into endocrine mechanisms, the microbiome, and genetic factors, future management will become more personalised. For now, a strong base of family-centred care, recognition of treatable endocrine causes, and judicious use of new therapies can reduce the burden of childhood obesity and its complications.

Abbreviations

ASMBS	American Society for Metabolic and Bariatric Surgery BMI:body mass index
CDC	Centers for Disease Control and Prevention
EDCs	endocrine-disrupting chemicals
GHD	growth hormone deficiency
GLP-1 RA	glucagon-like peptide-1 receptor agonist HbA1c: glycated haemoglobin
IFSO	International Federation for the Surgery of Obesity and Metabolic Disorders
IGF-1	insulin-like growth factor-1
LMICs	low- and middle-income countries MAFLD: metabolic-associated fatty liver disease MC4R: melanocortin 4 receptor
PCOS	polycystic ovary syndrome
POMC	proopiomelanocortin
WHO	World Health Organization

Acknowledgements

The authors acknowledge the use of Grammarly for grammar, spelling, punctuation, and language editing, as well as the use of ChatGPT for summarisation of author-generated content during the preparation of this book chapter. All content was independently reviewed and verified by the authors, who take full responsibility for the accuracy and integrity of the chapter.

Conflict of Interest

The authors declare no conflict of interest.

Author details

Harrison Samuel[1*] and Helen Harrison[2]

1 Department of Family Medicine, Asokoro District Hospital, Abuja, Nigeria

2 Kubwa General Hospital, Abuja, Nigeria

*Address all correspondence to: otuharrisonsamuel@gmail.com

IntechOpen

References

[1] World Health Organization. Obesity and overweight [Internet]. Geneva: WHO; 2025. Available from: https://www.who.int/news-room/fact-sheets/detail/obesity-and-overweight [Accessed: 2025-September-01]

[2] NCD Risk Factor Collaboration (NCD-RisC). Worldwide trends in underweight and obesity from 1990 to 2022: A pooled analysis of 3663 population-representative studies with 222 million children, adolescents, and adults. Lancet. 2024;**403**(10431): 1027–1050. DOI: 10.1016/S0140-6736(23)02750-2

[3] Kumar S, Kelly AS. Review of childhood obesity: From epidemiology, etiology, and comorbidities to clinical assessment and treatment. Mayo Clinic Proceedings. 2017;**92**(2):251–265. DOI: 10.1016/j.mayocp.2016.09.017

[4] Hemat Jouy HR, Beheshti F, Taghikhani M, et al. Adipokines in the crosstalk between adipose tissues and other organs: Implications in cardiometabolic diseases. Biomedicines. 2024;**12**(9):2129. DOI: 10.3390/biomedicines12092129

[5] Song K, Kim HS, Chae HW. Nonalcoholic fatty liver disease and insulin resistance in children. Clinical and Experimental Pediatrics. 2023;**66**(12):512–519. DOI: 10.3345/cep.2022.01312

[6] Hampl SE, Hassink SG, Skinner AC, et al. Clinical practice guideline for the evaluation and treatment of children and adolescents with obesity. Pediatrics. 2023;**151**(2):e2022060640. DOI: 10.1542/peds.2022-060640

[7] Dalamaga M, Kounatidis D, Tsilingiris D, et al. The role of endocrine disruptors bisphenols and phthalates in obesity: Current evidence, perspectives and controversies. International Journal of Molecular Sciences. 2024;**25**(1):675. DOI: 10.3390/ijms25010675

[8] Müller TD, Nogueiras R, Andermann ML, et al. Ghrelin. Molecular Metabolism. 2015; **4**(6):437–460. DOI: 10.1016/j.molmet.2015.03.005

[9] Styne DM, Arslanian SA, Connor EL, et al. Pediatric obesity-assessment, treatment, and prevention: An endocrine society clinical practice guideline. Journal of Clinical Endocrinology and Metabolism. 2017;**102**(3):709–757. DOI: 10.1210/jc.2016-2573

[10] Clément K, van den Akker E, Argente J, et al. Setmelanotide POMC and LEPR phase 3 trial investigators. Efficacy and safety of setmelanotide, an MC4R agonist, in individuals with severe obesity due to LEPR or POMC deficiency: Single-arm, open-label, multicentre, phase 3 trials. The Lancet Diabetes & Endocrinology. 2020;**8**(12):960–970. DOI: 10.1016/S2213-8587(20)30364-8

[11] Zigman JM, Bouret SG, Andrews ZB. Obesity impairs the action of the neuroendocrine ghrelin system. Trends in Endocrinology and Metabolism. 2016;**27**(1):54–63. DOI: 10.1016/j.tem.2015.09.010

[12] Chait A, den Hartigh LJ. Adipose tissue distribution, inflammation and its metabolic consequences, including diabetes and cardiovascular disease.

Frontiers in Cardiovascular Medicine. 2020;**7**:22. DOI: 10.3389/fcvm.2020.00022

[13] Francisco V, Pino J, Campos-Cabaleiro V, et al. Obesity, fat mass and immune system: Role for leptin. Frontiers in Physiology. 2018;**9**:640

[14] Reinehr T, Roth CL. Inflammation markers in type 2 diabetes and the metabolic syndrome in the pediatric population. Current Diabetes Reports. 2018;**18**(12):131. DOI: 10.1007/s11892-018-1110-5

[15] Hu W, Zhu H, Gong F. Leptin and leptin resistance in obesity: Current evidence, mechanisms and future directions. Endocrine Connections. 2025;**14**(9):e250521. DOI: 10.1530/EC-25-0521

[16] Hawton K, Shirodkar D, Siese T, et al. A recent update on childhood obesity: Aetiology, treatment and complications. Journal of Pediatric Endocrinology and Metabolism. 2025;**38**(5):429–441. DOI: 10.1515/jpem-2024-0316

[17] Vos MB, Abrams SH, Barlow SE, et al. NASPGHAN clinical practice guideline for the diagnosis and treatment of nonalcoholic fatty liver disease in children: Recommendations from the expert committee on NAFLD (ECON) and the North American Society of Pediatric Gastroenterology. Hepatology and Nutrition (NASPGHAN). 2017;**64**(2):319–334. DOI: 10.1097/MPG.0000000000001482

[18] Malavolta E, Cammisa I, Rotunno G, et al. The Impact of Acquired Hypothyroidism on the Growth and Metabolic Profiles of Pediatric Patients: A Retrospective Monocentric Study. Children (Basel). 2025;**12**(3):272. DOI: 10.3390/children12030272

[19] Ferruzzi A, Vrech M, Pietrobelli A, et al. The influence of growth hormone on pediatric body composition: A systematic review. Frontiers in Endocrinology (Lausanne). 2023;**14**:1093691. DOI: 10.3389/fendo.2023.1093691

[20] Forcina G, Di Filippo P, De Biasio D, et al. Targeting the gut microbiota in pediatric obesity: A paradigm shift in prevention and treatment? A comprehensive review. Nutrients. 2025;**17**(18):2942. DOI: 10.3390/nu17182942

[21] Mainieri F, La Bella S, Rinaldi M, et al. Rare genetic forms of obesity in childhood and adolescence, a comprehensive review of their molecular mechanisms and diagnostic approach. European Journal of Pediatrics. 2023;**182**(11):4781–4793. DOI: 10.1007/s00431-023-05159-x

[22] Pomahacova R, Paterova P, Nykodymova E, et al. Overweight and obesity in children and adolescents with endocrine disorders. Biomed Papers of the Medical Faculty of the University Palacky Olomouc Czech Republic. 2023;**167**(4):328–334. DOI: 10.5507/bp.2023.036

[23] Badr M, El-Rabaa G, Freiha M, Niechciał E, et al. Endocrine consequences of childhood obesity: A narrative review. Frontiers in Endocrinology (Lausanne. 2025;**16**:1584861. DOI: 10.3389/fendo.2025.1584861

[24] Weghuber D, Barrett T, Barrientos-Pérez M, et al. STEP TEENS investigators. Once-weekly semaglutide

in adolescents with obesity. The New England Journal of Medicine. 2022;**387**(24):2245–2257. DOI: 10.1056/NEJMoa2208601

[25] Haliloglu B, Bereket A. Hypothalamic obesity in children: Pathophysiology to clinical management. Journal of Pediatric Endocrinology and Metabolism. 2015;**28**(5-6):503–513. DOI: 10.1515/jpem-2014-0512

[26] Kühnen P, Clément K, Wiegand S, et al. Proopiomelanocortin deficiency treated with a melanocortin-4 receptor agonist. The New England Journal of Medicine. 2016;**375**(3):240–246. DOI: 10.1056/NEJMoa1512693

[27] Whitehead L, Kabdebo I, Dunham M, et al. The effectiveness of nurse-led interventions to prevent childhood and adolescent overweight and obesity: A systematic review of randomised trials. Journal of Advanced Nursing. 2021;**77**(12):4612–4631. DOI: 10.1111/jan.14928

[28] Guerra Toro HI, Jaramillo AP, Caceres VM. Family-based interventions for pediatric obesity: A comprehensive systematic review and meta-analysis of their effectiveness. Cureus. 2024;**16**(8):e65919. DOI: 10.7759/cureus.65919

[29] Ahmed U, Mahmood MS, Parsons M, et al. A systematic review looking at the current best practices as well as primary care practitioner's views on the diagnosis and treatment of childhood obesity. Cureus. 2023;**15**(1):e34346. DOI: 10.7759/cureus.34346

[30] Sethi AK, Velarambath Manalil S, Das S, et al. Quality improvement initiative to standardise the anthropometric assessment for children under the age of 5 years at an urban primary health centre in New Delhi. BMJ Open Quality. 2024;**13**(2):e002583. DOI: 10.1136/bmjoq-2023-002583

[31] Kelly AS, Auerbach P, Barrientos-Perez M, et al. A randomized, controlled trial of liraglutide for adolescents with obesity. The New England Journal of Medicine. 2020;**382**(22):2117–2128. DOI: 10.1056/NEJMoa1916038

[32] Fox CK, Barrientos-Pérez M, Bomberg EM, et al. Liraglutide for children 6 to <12 years of age with obesity-a randomized trial. The New England Journal of Medicine. 2025;**392**(6):555–565. DOI: 10.1056/NEJMoa2407379

[33] Brown RJ, Meehan CA, Cochran E, et al. Effects of metreleptin in pediatric patients with lipodystrophy. Journal of Clinical Endocrinology and Metabolism. 2017;**102**(5):1511–1519. DOI: 10.1210/jc.2016-3628

[34] Pratt JSA, Browne A, Browne NT, et al. ASMBS pediatric metabolic and bariatric surgery guidelines, 2018. Surgery for Obesity and Related Diseases. 2018;**14**(7):882–901. DOI: 10.1016/j.soard.2018.03.019

Section 3

PCOS/PMOS (Polyendocrine Metabolic Ovarian Syndrome)

Chapter 4

When Periods Go Missing: Recognizing PCOS Early in Youth

Irasema Apodaca-Ramos and Cynthia Ruiz-Carranza

Abstract

Polycystic ovary syndrome (PCOS) is one of the most common endocrine disorders in adolescents, yet its diagnosis during this developmental stage remains particularly challenging. Pubertal physiology overlaps with early manifestations of PCOS, often delaying recognition and treatment. The condition arises from a multifactorial pathophysiology involving genetic predisposition, ovarian and neuroendocrine dysfunction, insulin resistance, and environmental influences. Clinically, adolescents may present with irregular menstrual cycles persisting beyond two years postmenarche, acne, hirsutism, or biochemical hyperandrogenism. Unlike in adults, ultrasound findings and anti-Müllerian hormone levels should not be used for diagnosis in this age group, as multifollicular ovaries are common during normal puberty. PCOS not only impacts reproductive health but also carries long-term metabolic risks, including insulin resistance, obesity, dyslipidemia, and increased lifetime risk of type 2 diabetes and cardiovascular disease. Psychological effects such as depression, anxiety, and body image concerns are frequent and must be integrated into care. Management strategies emphasize lifestyle interventions, cycle regulation with combined oral contraceptives, consideration of metformin in selected cases, and targeted dermatologic or psychological support. A multidisciplinary, individualized, and stigma-free approach is essential to optimize outcomes. Early recognition, family-centered counseling, and longitudinal follow-up are key to preventing misdiagnosis, supporting adolescent well-being, and reducing the long-term cardiometabolic burden of the syndrome.

Keywords: polycystic ovary syndrome, menstrual irregularities, pediatric and adolescent gynecology, early diagnosis, hormonal disorders

1. Introduction

> *Ana, 16, enjoys playing soccer but has recently avoided practice due to concerns about her skin. Despite trying multiple creams, her severe acne persists. She also feels embarrassed by the development of new facial hair on her upper lip. Her periods are unpredictable – sometimes occurring every six weeks, other times skipping for up to three months. When she and her mom visit the clinic, their main concern is whether*

this is just "normal teenage stuff" or something that needs medical attention.

Menstrual irregularities during adolescence are among the most common reasons for gynecologic consultation. While variability in menstrual cycles is expected in the first years following menarche, persistent amenorrhea or oligomenorrhea should prompt careful evaluation. Polycystic ovary syndrome (PCOS) is a widespread disorder with endocrine–metabolic impairment in women of reproductive age. The condition arises from a multifactorial pathophysiology that includes genetic predisposition, primary ovarian dysfunction, neuroendocrine alterations, and metabolic susceptibility. Contributing factors such as insulin resistance (IR), hyperinsulinemia, obesity, and changes in adipokines like adiponectin further complicate the clinical picture [1].

The clinical manifestations of PCOS are diverse, but the most commonly observed are acne, hirsutism, persistent menstrual irregularities beyond two years after menarche, and clinical or biochemical hyperandrogenism. The diagnosis of PCOS in adolescents requires careful consideration of clinical features and the exclusion of other conditions [2–4].

Diagnosis is established using criteria that include chronic anovulation and elevated androgen levels. Unlike in adult patients, the use of pelvic ultrasound is not recommended in this age group due to the high prevalence of polycystic morphology as a result of normal pubertal development [5].

Beyond reproductive manifestations, PCOS is associated with a range of metabolic complications. These include IR, impaired glucose tolerance, obesity, dyslipidemia, and infertility. Such consequences are thought to result from disruptions in pituitary hormone secretion, ovarian folliculogenesis, and insulin signaling pathways. Management in adolescents requires particular care, especially regarding the transition into adulthood and the impact on fertility [2–4].

PCOS in adolescents presents unique diagnostic and management challenges. The overlapping features of normal pubertal development and early manifestations of PCOS often lead to uncertainty, delayed recognition, or even misdiagnosis. This chapter aims to guide clinicians toward a clear understanding of the condition in this age group. The objectives are threefold: first, to improve early recognition of PCOS by highlighting its distinct clinical and biochemical features during adolescence; second, to prevent misdiagnosis through careful differentiation between physiologic pubertal changes and pathological findings; and third, to emphasize the long-term health implications of PCOS, including reproductive, metabolic, and psychological outcomes. By addressing these objectives, the chapter underscores the importance of timely, accurate, and holistic care for adolescents at risk of or living with PCOS.

2. Physiology of normal pubertal development

Puberty represents the transitional stage between childhood and the acquisition of reproductive capacity. While it is often defined as the biological process of sexual maturation, a broader perspective places puberty within the context of adolescence. This expanded view encourages healthcare providers to also consider the psychological, behavioral, and social dimensions that accompany physical pubertal changes [6].

The hypothalamic-pituitary-gonadal (HPG) axis plays a central role in driving the physical changes of puberty. A key step in this process is the shift from continuous to pulsatile secretion of gonadotropin-releasing hormone (GnRH) by the hypothalamus. This pulsatility stimulates the anterior pituitary to release luteinizing hormone (LH) and follicle-stimulating hormone (FSH), which, in turn, promote the production of estradiol in the ovaries [7].

The estradiol produced by the ovaries is a key driver of pubertal development; it contributes to breast growth, genital changes, and bone maturation, with these estrogen-mediated changes occurring in a stepwise sequence [7].

Thelarche, or the beginning of breast development, is usually the first visible sign of puberty in females, generally appearing between ages 8.8 and 10, though timing may differ across racial and ethnic groups. Adrenarche, marked by the growth of pubic hair, tends to occur around the same age range. Soon after, the pubertal growth spurt begins, with an average onset at 9.5 years and peak growth velocity near 11.5 years. Menarche typically follows at about 12.5 years, after which additional height gain is limited, averaging 2–2.5 years with less than 5 cm of further growth [7].

Menarche marks the culmination of pubertal maturation and reflects the functional activation of the hypothalamic-pituitary-ovarian (HPO) axis. The timing of menarche is influenced by genetic, metabolic, and environmental factors, with kisspeptin signaling playing a critical role in GnRH activation. Although menarche signifies the onset of reproductive potential, ovulatory cycles are often irregular in the first years due to the immaturity of the HPO axis, gradually progressing toward the regular, coordinated cycles of adulthood [8].

So, what is normal in adolescence? As mentioned before, menstrual periods are often irregular in adolescents after menarche due to the immaturity of the HPO axis, particularly the delayed maturation of estrogen's positive feedback on LH. During the first two years postmenarche, 50–80% of cycles are anovulatory, and even up to five years later, 10–20% of cycles may remain anovulatory. Over time, cycle regularity improves, with most adolescents achieving a pattern of 21–45 days (average 32). The pace of this transition is influenced by the age of menarche; those with earlier menarche tend to reach ovulatory cycles sooner than those with later onset. Normal menstrual blood loss averages around 40 ml per cycle (range 25–69 ml), with volumes >80 ml considered heavy menstrual bleeding (HMB). Importantly, HMB at menarche may be the first sign of an underlying bleeding disorder, which accounts for up to 20% of adolescents presenting with this complaint, highlighting the need for careful evaluation [7].

3. Defining PCOS in adolescents

Because puberty involves many physiological changes (irregular cycles, acne, changing hormone levels), diagnosing PCOS in adolescents can be a challenge, leading to delayed diagnosis and treatment. Current guidelines (Pediatric Endocrine Society, Endocrine Society 2018, International PCOS Guideline 2023) recommend that two main features must be met [9–11] (See **Appendix A**).

- Irregular menstrual cycles (ovulatory dysfunction)
  - o Patterns in cycle irregularity are assessed in relation to the duration since menarche.
  - o In the one to two years postmenarche, irregular cycles are common and physiologic. By the third postmenarche year, about 95% of those assigned female at birth have cycle lengths within the adult range (21–45 days). Persistent cycles outside this range after that point may suggest dysfunction.
- Clinical or biochemical hyperandrogenism
  - o Clinical: hirsutism, moderate-to-severe acne, and/or androgenic alopecia. Mild acne is common in adolescents and is not necessarily abnormal.
  - o Biochemical: elevated androgens in blood tests.
    - o Free testosterone or the free androgen index (FAI) offers the best sensitivity/specificity.
    - o Total testosterone, androstenedione, and DHEA are less specific [12].

It is a requirement that adolescent PCOS should be diagnosed only when ovulatory dysfunction and hyperandrogenism persist >2 years postmenarche, after excluding mimicking conditions such as thyroid disease, hyperprolactinemia, nonclassical congenital adrenal hyperplasia, androgen-secreting tumors, and exogenous androgen use [12].

To avoid overdiagnosis, it is worth mentioning and emphasizing that polycystic ovarian morphology on ultrasound should not be used in adolescents (at least the first eight years postmenarche), as multifollicular ovaries are common during normal puberty [13]. Neither are anti-Müllerian hormone levels suitable for diagnosis due to their limited variability in assays and overlap with normal development.

Adolescents who have only one of the required features are considered “at risk” for PCOS and should be monitored longitudinally, with attention to symptom progression, metabolic screening, lifestyle factors, etc.

4. Epidemiology and risk factors

Global prevalence of PCOS in adolescents’ estimates varies with the diagnostic criteria applied, but recent adolescent meta-analyses and the International Evidence-Based Guideline place adolescent prevalence in the low-to-mid single digits to 10%, with higher estimates when adult Rotterdam-type criteria are used. Lower, approximately 6%, when using adolescent-aware international guideline criteria.

Incident rates peak during mid-to-late adolescence, between 15 and 19 years, when ovulatory dysfunction and hyperandrogenism become more apparent [14].

The prevalence varies by region and by the population sampled (school-based vs. clinic-based cohorts); differences likely reflect true variation plus methodological heterogeneity.

4.1 Risk factors

PCOS in adolescence is strongly associated with obesity, IR, and a family history of PCOS/androgen excess; prenatal androgen exposure, early rapid weight gain, and certain environmental exposures are candidate upstream drivers. Early identification of at-risk girls permits targeted counseling and metabolic surveillance (See **Appendix B**).

- Obesity is the strongest modifiable risk factor, the most consistently reported correlate, and an apparent amplifier of the PCOS phenotype in adolescents. Higher childhood and peripubertal BMI and central adiposity are associated with later hyperandrogenism, oligo-anovulation, and metabolic dysfunction. Mechanistically, adiposity promotes IR, hyperinsulinemia, and altered steroid metabolism – each of which augments ovarian androgen production and reduces hepatic sex-hormone-binding globulin (SHBG), thereby increasing free androgens. Several longitudinal and cross-sectional studies and reviews document these links [15].

- IR is common in adolescent PCOS, even among nonobese individuals assigned female at birth, and it amplifies ovarian androgen secretion while reducing SHBG. IR is both a mediator (linking adiposity to hyperandrogenism) and an independent trait in familial PCOS predisposition. Clinical implication: screening for IR-related metabolic features should begin in adolescents with suspected PCOS [16].

- PCOS shows familial clustering. Genome-wide association studies highlight polygenic susceptibility, particularly in pathways of gonadotropin secretion, insulin signaling, and androgen biosynthesis. Mendelian randomization and genetic studies suggest genetic liability overlaps with metabolic pathways and androgen biosynthesis. A family history of PCOS or early-onset metabolic disease elevates risk [17].

- Prenatal androgen exposure, maternal PCOS, and in utero metabolic dysfunction may "program" susceptibility in offspring. This developmental origin hypothesis is supported by translational models and human cohort studies. Evidence is growing, but causal pathways in humans are still under active investigation [18].

- Early menarche, rapid prepubertal weight gain, sedentary lifestyle, and diets that promote adiposity are linked to a higher risk of PCOS. These peripubertal windows are critical because the neuroendocrine changes of puberty can reveal an underlying predisposition [19].

- Emerging data suggest that endocrine-disrupting chemicals, heavy metals, and other pollutants may contribute to PCOS pathogenesis; results are heterogeneous, and causality is unproven [20]. This remains an important research area.

Early recognition of risk factors allows targeted counseling and prevention of long-term metabolic sequelae. Adolescents with obesity, a family history of PCOS, or persistent menstrual irregularities should undergo assessment for hyperandrogenism and metabolic risk.

5. Clinical features in adolescents

Irregular menstrual cycles are common during the first year after menarche as part of the pubertal transition. However, beyond this period, certain patterns are considered abnormal: cycles shorter than 21 days or longer than 45 days between one and three-years postmenarche; cycles shorter than 21 days, longer than 35 days, or fewer than eight cycles per year more than three years postmenarche until perimenopause; any cycle lasting more than 90 days more than one year after menarche; or primary amenorrhea by age 15 or more than three years after thelarche. When these abnormalities are present, PCOS should be considered according to guideline recommendations.

Adolescents may present with additional clinical features, such as:

- Hyperandrogenic symptoms: moderate-to-severe acne, hirsutism, and occasionally androgenic alopecia.
- Obesity or weight gain, which may exacerbate metabolic and reproductive features.
- Psychosocial and emotional concerns, including distress about body image, acne, and hirsutism, contribute to increased rates of depression and anxiety.

Because clinical signs of PCOS can overlap with normal puberty, particularly in the first two years postmenarche, adolescents who exhibit features but do not yet meet diagnostic criteria may be considered "at increased risk." These individuals should be followed over time, especially if symptoms persist or significant weight gain occurs during adolescence.

6. Diagnostic work-up

A structured diagnostic work-up is essential to differentiate physiologic pubertal changes from PCOS in adolescents. Evaluation should begin with a detailed history of menstrual patterns relative to years postmenarche, the onset and progression of symptoms, and family history of PCOS, diabetes, or early cardiovascular disease. On physical examination, clinicians should record BMI, waist circumference, and blood pressure, and document clinical signs of androgen excess such as hirsutism, moderate-to-severe acne, or androgenic alopecia (See **Appendix C**).

Biochemical testing should prioritize total and free testosterone, or the FAI, as first-line markers of hyperandrogenism. Targeted exclusion of mimickers is required, including 17-hydroxyprogesterone (to rule out nonclassic congenital adrenal hyperplasia [NCCAH]), TSH (for thyroid disease), and prolactin (for hyperprolactinemia). When androgen results are inconclusive, androstenedione or dehydroepiandrosterone sulfate (DHEAS) may be measured, although these are less specific and decline with age. Markedly elevated androgen levels beyond the reference range should always prompt consideration of alternative causes, such as androgen-secreting tumors. Clinical hirsutism may be quantified with the Ferriman-Gallwey score, though ethnic and developmental variations must be considered. Pelvic ultrasound should not be used for diagnosis in adolescents within eight years of menarche, given the high prevalence of multifollicular ovaries during normal puberty and the absence of validated criteria for this age group.

Because PCOS carries significant metabolic implications, comprehensive cardiometabolic screening is recommended at the time of diagnosis. A fasting lipid profile – including total cholesterol, low-density lipoprotein (LDL), high-density lipoprotein (HDL), and triglycerides – should be obtained, with repeat testing individualized according to baseline results and comorbidities. In addition to cardiovascular risk, adolescents with PCOS have a substantially increased risk of impaired glucose tolerance and type 2 diabetes mellitus, largely driven by intrinsic IR and β-cell dysfunction. This risk is evident even among those with normal body mass index, underscoring that obesity is an aggravating but not necessary factor. Current international guidelines recommend that glycemic status in all individuals with PCOS should be assessed using a 75-gram oral glucose tolerance test (OGTT), which remains the most sensitive tool for detecting early dysglycemia. In contrast, fasting glucose and HbA1c alone have limited sensitivity and may miss up to 40% of cases of impaired glucose tolerance. Repeat OGTT screening is advised every one to three years, with frequency individualized according to baseline results, BMI, family history, and other risk factors.

Although IR is central to PCOS pathophysiology, available clinical assays for fasting insulin or homeostasis model assessment (HOMA-IR) have poor reproducibility and limited clinical utility and, therefore, are not recommended for routine diagnosis or monitoring. Instead, emphasis should be placed on systematic glycemic testing and early intervention when abnormalities are detected. These steps align with international PCOS guidelines and adolescent-specific recommendations, which emphasize requiring both menstrual irregularity (by years postmenarche) and clinical or biochemical hyperandrogenism, while deferring polycystic ovarian morphology as a diagnostic criterion in early postmenarcheal years (see **Figure 1**).

7. Differential diagnosis

Menstrual irregularity and hyperandrogenic signs in early adolescence often overlap with normal pubertal physiology, so a structured differential is essential (**Table 1**). First, consider physiologic pubertal anovulation in the first years after menarche; cyclic irregularity can be normal during maturation of the HPO axis and should be interpreted against years postmenarche before labeling PCOS [21]. Screen for functional hypothalamic amenorrhea (FHA) when there is weight loss, high exercise load, psychosocial stress, or low energy availability – look for low/normal gonadotropins and estradiol after excluding pregnancy and other

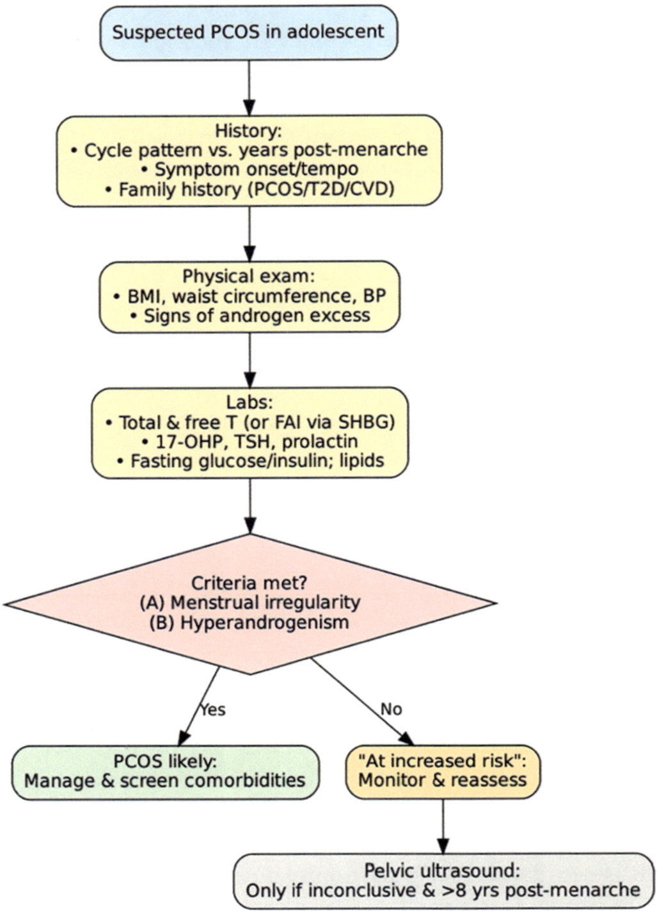

Figure 1.
Diagnostic work-up for teen AFAB (generated with AI help).

causes [22]. Evaluate hyperprolactinemia in the presence of galactorrhea, headaches/visual symptoms, or amenorrhea with low gonadotropins; confirm with a fasting prolactin and review drugs that raise prolactin [23]. Check for thyroid dysfunction in any menstrual disorder (TSH ± free T4), as both hypo and hyperthyroidism can alter bleeding patterns [24]. Exclude NCCAH with an early-morning 17-hydroxyprogesterone (± ACTH stimulation when borderline), especially in hyperandrogenic teens or those with early pubarche [25]. Finally, keep rare but important causes in mind: Cushing's syndrome (progressive weight gain with stunting of growth velocity, purple striae, proximal myopathy) and androgen-secreting tumors (rapidly progressive hirsutism/virilization, very high androgens); these warrant expedited referral [26]. Throughout, apply adolescent-specific PCOS guidance (irregular cycles defined by years postmenarche; requirement for clinical/biochemical hyperandrogenism; ultrasound not recommended for diagnosis ≤8 years postmenarche) [27].

DOI: http://dx.doi.org/10.5772/intechopen.1013810

Condition	When to suspect (history/exam)	First-line tests	Clues distinguishing from PCOS	Next steps/referral
Physiologic pubertal anovulation	First 1–3 yrs postmenarche: irregular cycles without significant hyperandrogenism; normal growth/puberty trajectory.	Pregnancy test as indicated; observation with cycle tracking.	Timing relative to menarche; typically mild acne; symptoms often normalize with time. Ultrasound not for diagnosis <8 years postmenarche.	Reassess over time; provide lifestyle counseling; avoid premature PCOS labeling.
Functional hypothalamic amenorrhea (FHA)	Low energy availability, weight loss, high training load, stress; often bradycardia, low BMI, or recent weight change.	β-hCG; FSH/LH; estradiol; TSH; prolactin; CBC/electrolytes, if indicated.	Low/normal gonadotropins and estradiol; improvement with nutritional/behavioral restoration; no biochemical hyperandrogenism.	Refer to adolescent medicine/endocrinology; multidisciplinary nutrition-psychology support.
Hyperprolactinemia	Galactorrhea, headaches/visual field changes; amenorrhea/oligomenorrhea; medications that raise prolactin.	Fasting prolactin (repeat to confirm), TSH, pregnancy test, medication review.	Low/normal gonadotropins; androgen levels not elevated unless cocondition is present.	If prolactin levels are persistently high or very elevated, pituitary imaging and an endocrine referral are recommended.
Thyroid dysfunction (hypo-/hyper-)	Fatigue, weight changes, cold/heat intolerance, hair/skin changes; menstrual irregularity spectrum from amenorrhea to menorrhagia.	TSH ± free T4 (consider TPOAb if hypothyroid).	Menstrual abnormalities resolve with thyroid correction; no primary hyperandrogenism.	Treat per thyroid guidelines; consult pediatric endocrinology if uncertain.
Nonclassic congenital adrenal hyperplasia (21-hydroxylase deficiency)	Early pubarche, accelerated growth/advanced bone age, hirsutism/acne; family/ethnic risk.	Early-morning 17-hydroxyprogesterone; ACTH stimulation if borderline.	Elevated 17-OHP (basal or post-ACTH); may mimic PCOS but starts earlier and often shows growth or bone age changes.	Endocrinology referral for confirmation and management.
Cushing's syndrome (rare)	Progressive truncal obesity with **poor linear growth**, purple striae, easy bruising, proximal muscle weakness, and hypertension.	Initial screening: late-night salivary cortisol, 1-mg DST, or 24-h UFC (per guideline).	Catabolic stigmata and growth deceleration distinguish it from PCOS; cortisol tests are abnormal.	Urgent endocrine referral; imaging to localize the source.
Androgen-secreting tumor (ovarian/adrenal; rare)	**Rapid-onset** hirsutism/virilization (deep voice, clitoromegaly), very high testosterone or DHEAS, symptoms progressing despite therapy.	Total testosterone, SHBG → FAI; DHEAS; ± androstenedione. If markedly elevated, urgent imaging (pelvic US/MRI; adrenal CT/MRI).	Abrupt course and **marked** androgen elevations, unlike typical PCOS.	**Expedited** referral to endocrinology, gynecology oncology, or urology for work-up and treatment.

Notes for application in teens: Use adolescent-specific PCOS criteria (irregular cycles defined by years postmenarche; require hyperandrogenism; defer ovarian morphology for diagnosis until >8 years postmenarche). Apply shared decision-making, avoid premature "infertility" labeling, and reassess longitudinally when findings are equivocal [4].

Table1.
Differential diagnosis [4].

8. Management strategies

Lifestyle intervention remains the cornerstone of management in adolescents with PCOS. A structured approach that combines exercise, dietary strategies, and behavioral support should be recommended to all affected individuals, as it can improve metabolic health, reduce central adiposity, and optimize lipid profiles. Importantly, healthcare professionals should emphasize that the benefits of healthy lifestyle changes extend beyond weight loss, supporting cardiometabolic health even in adolescents with a normal BMI. Early engagement in sustainable lifestyle behaviors also facilitates long-term adherence and reduces the risk of developing IR, type 2 diabetes, and cardiovascular disease, which are heightened in this population [4] (See **Appendix D**).

8.1 Pharmacological therapy is considered in symptom-driven and risk-based contexts

Combined oral contraceptives (COCPs) may be offered to adolescents with PCOS, or those at risk, to regulate menstrual cycles and address hyperandrogenic symptoms such as hirsutism and acne. Prescribing should follow a shared decision-making model, including education on efficacy, safety, contraindications, and the need for individualized choices regarding estrogen dose and formulation. Metformin may be considered, particularly in adolescents with overweight/obesity or metabolic risk, with gradual dose titration and use of extended-release preparations to minimize side effects; however, evidence in this age group remains limited. Anti-obesity agents (e.g., liraglutide, semaglutide, or orlistat) are not first-line but could be considered in severe weight-related cases following general population guidelines, with gradual escalation for GLP-1 agonists to reduce gastrointestinal intolerance. Antiandrogen medications such as spironolactone may be used as adjunct therapy for persistent hirsutism, although safety and risk profiles (e.g., liver toxicity with finasteride, flutamide, or bicalutamide, and meningioma risk with high-dose cyproterone acetate) require careful discussion. Finally, inositol supplementation may be considered based on patient preference, with potential metabolic benefits but limited impact on clinical outcomes such as ovulation or hirsutism [4].

8.2 Dermatology referral (severe acne/hirsutism)

Severe, scarring, or treatment-refractory acne in adolescents with suspected or confirmed PCOS warrants early dermatology comanagement to optimize outcomes and consider isotretinoin when appropriate; similarly, moderate-to-severe hirsutism that impairs quality of life or fails first-line measures benefits from dermatologic and/or endocrine input for multimodal therapy (pharmacologic + hair-removal methods). Current acne guidelines from the American Academy of Dermatology endorse escalation to systemic therapies (including isotretinoin with appropriate monitoring) for severe or refractory disease, while hirsutism guidance from the Endocrine Society emphasizes evaluation for androgen excess and patient-important treatment combining antiandrogens/COCs with direct hair-reduction techniques [28, 29].

DOI: http://dx.doi.org/10.5772/intechopen.1013810

8.3 Psychological support (screening and counseling)

Adolescents with PCOS have a substantially higher prevalence of depressive symptoms, and guidelines recommend routine, age-appropriate screening for depression (and consideration of anxiety), followed by timely referral for counseling or psychological therapies when positive. The 2023 International PCOS Guideline and its adolescent summary report a up to four-fold higher prevalence of depression in adolescents with PCOS versus peers, and call for ongoing rescreening based on clinical judgment and life changes; they also highlight frequent reports from teens that their concerns are minimized, underscoring the need for empathetic communication and shared decision-making [12].

8.4 Individualized care – avoid premature "infertility" labeling

In adolescents, diagnostic uncertainty is common (e.g., physiologic anovulation, mild acne), and guidelines caution against premature labeling – particularly around "infertility" – which may increase distress without informing immediate care. The adolescent recommendations from the 2023 International PCOS Guideline advocate framing many youths with only one diagnostic feature as "at risk," focusing care on present symptoms (cycles, dermatologic concerns, metabolic risk), longitudinal follow-up, and supportive education rather than future infertility; this approach is associated with better engagement and addresses frequent dissatisfaction when visits focus primarily on fertility rather than current needs [12].

9. Patient and family education

Effective patient and family education is central to optimizing outcomes in adolescents with PCOS. Communication should be clear, respectful, and free of stigma, using plain, developmentally appropriate language. The diagnosis should be named only when criteria are fully met or when the adolescent is considered "at risk." In these conversations, a shared-decision framework (e.g., SPIKE) is recommended to guide how PCOS is explained – clarifying what the condition is, and, equally important, what it is not. The 2023 International Evidence-Based PCOS Guideline highlights the importance of respectful dialogue, shared decision-making with both adolescents and caregivers, and the use of validated educational resources to support knowledge and self-management [4].

Addressing stigma is essential, as misconceptions are common and strongly associated with poorer well-being.

Adolescents frequently report distress related to weight, acne, hirsutism, and body image, underscoring the need for empathetic counseling and normalization [30]. One critical misconception to correct is the belief that PCOS inevitably causes infertility. Most patients will eventually ovulate spontaneously or with simple interventions when pregnancy is desired. In adolescence, the primary focus should remain on symptom management and prevention of long-term metabolic complications rather than future fertility [30].

Adolescent-friendly resources, peer support, and digital tools can strengthen education and engagement. Vetted, youth-appropriate material and safe peer/community support options empower patients to manage their condition beyond the clinical setting. Evidence-based digital tools, such as the AskPCOS app – developed in line with international guidelines and codesigned with patients – have demonstrated effectiveness as trusted sources of information. Reviews of PCOS-related apps suggest growing quality and potential benefits for lifestyle change and self-management, particularly when recommended and curated by clinicians [31].

Finally, despite advances in understanding PCOS, important gaps remain. Reliable diagnostic biomarkers are still lacking, adolescent-specific hormonal thresholds are limited, and few longitudinal studies exist to describe the natural history from puberty into adulthood. Early recognition and intervention remain critical to reducing the long-term cardiometabolic burden of PCOS, including the risks of IR, type 2 diabetes, and cardiovascular disease. Optimal care requires a multidisciplinary model, integrating pediatrics, gynecology, endocrinology, nutrition, and psychology to provide individualized support for both physical and emotional health in adolescents with PCOS.

10. Conclusion

PCOS in adolescents represents a complex condition where physiologic pubertal changes overlap with pathological features, creating unique diagnostic and management challenges. Evidence-based practice requires careful application of adolescent-specific criteria, avoidance of premature labeling, and a focus on addressing present symptoms while monitoring long-term risks. Early, individualized interventions – centered on lifestyle modification, menstrual regulation, and metabolic screening – can mitigate future reproductive and cardiometabolic complications. Multidisciplinary collaboration and sensitive communication with patients and families are essential to reduce stigma, dispel myths such as the equation of PCOS with infertility, and empower adolescents toward lifelong self-management. Ongoing research into diagnostic biomarkers, hormonal cutoffs, and longitudinal outcomes will be critical to refining care, but current best practice emphasizes early recognition, holistic management, and adolescent-centered support as the foundation for improving outcomes across the lifespan.

Nomenclature

PCOS	Polycystic Ovary Syndrome
HPO axis	Hypothalamic–Pituitary–Ovarian axis
HPG axis	Hypothalamic–Pituitary–Gonadal axis
GnRH	Gonadotropin-Releasing Hormone
LH	Luteinizing Hormone
FSH	Follicle-Stimulating Hormone
SHBG	Sex Hormone-Binding Globulin
FAI	Free Androgen Index
DHEAS	Dehydroepiandrosterone Sulfate
NCCAH	Nonclassic Congenital Adrenal Hyperplasia
TSH	Thyroid-Stimulating Hormone
17-OHP	17-Hydroxyprogesterone
BMI	Body Mass Index

DOI: http://dx.doi.org/10.5772/intechopen.1013810

IR	Insulin Resistance
COCP	Combined Oral Contraceptive Pill
OGTT	Oral Glucose Tolerance Test
DST	Dexamethasone Suppression Test
UFC	Urinary Free Cortisol
HMB	Heavy Menstrual Bleeding

Appendices and nomenclature

Appendix A. Diagnostic criteria for PCOS in adolescents [9–11]

Requires both:

- Persistent ovulatory dysfunction (cycles outside the age-appropriate range >2 years postmenarche).

- Clinical or biochemical hyperandrogenism.

Exclude mimicking conditions (thyroid dysfunction, hyperprolactinemia, NCCAH, Cushing's, androgen-secreting tumors, exogenous androgen use).

Ultrasound and AMH levels are not recommended for diagnosis ≤8 years postmenarche.

Appendix B. Risk factors summary [15–20]

Strongest: obesity, IR, and family history of PCOS.

Others: prenatal androgen exposure, early menarche, rapid weight gain, sedentary lifestyle, dietary factors, endocrine-disrupting chemicals.

Appendix C. Clinical work-up template [4]

- History: menstrual cycle pattern, age at menarche, onset of acne/hirsutism, and family history of PCOS or metabolic disease.

- Physical exam: BMI, waist circumference, blood pressure, hirsutism scoring, and acne severity.

- Laboratory tests: total and free testosterone (or FAI), 17-OHP, TSH, prolactin, fasting glucose, and lipid profile.

- Imaging: pelvic ultrasound only if >8 years postmenarche and the diagnosis remains unclear.

Appendix D. Management framework [4, 12, 28, 29]

- Lifestyle: exercise, dietary counseling, and behavioral support.

- Pharmacologic: COCPs, metformin, spironolactone (case-specific), inositol.
- Referral: dermatology for severe acne/hirsutism.
- Psychology: mental health support.
- Education: emphasize that PCOS ≠ infertility; provide adolescent-friendly resources and apps (e.g., AskPCOS).

Author details

Irasema Apodaca-Ramos* and Cynthia Ruiz-Carranza
Tecnológico de Monterrey, Mexico City, Mexico

*Address all correspondence to: irasema.apra@gmail.com

References

[1] American Academy of Pediatrics. Equitable and Inclusive Care in Pediatrics: A Compendium of AAP Clinical Practice Guidelines and Policies. Itasca, IL, USA: American Academy of Pediatrics; 2024. 241 p

[2] Rosenfield RL. Current concepts of polycystic ovary syndrome pathogenesis. Current Opinion in Pediatrics. 2020;**32**(5):698–706

[3] Saleh FL, Starkman H, Furness A, Pfeifer SM, Kives S. Polycystic ovary syndrome in adolescents. Obstetrics and Gynecology Clinics of North America. 2024;**51**(4):679–693

[4] Teede HJ, et al. Recommendations from the 2023 international evidence-based guideline for the assessment and management of polycystic ovary syndrome. Human Reproduction. 2023;**38**:1655–1679

[5] Joham AE, Peña AS. Polycystic ovary syndrome in adolescence. Seminars in Reproductive Medicine. 2022;**40**(1-2):e1–e8

[6] Sanfilippo JS, Lara-Torre E, Edmonds DK, Templeman C, editors. Clinical Pediatric and Adolescent Gynecology. London: Informa Medical; 2009

[7] De Silva N, Tyson NA. NASPAG Essentials of Pediatric and Adolescent Gynecology. London: Churchill Livingstone; 2024

[8] Lacroix AE, Gondal H, Shumway KR, et al. Physiology, Menarche. In: StatPearls. Treasure Island (FL): StatPearls Publishing; 2026. https://www.ncbi.nlm.nih.gov/books/NBK470216/

[9] Teede H, Tay CT, Azziz R. Response to letter to the editor from Rosenfield et al. Recommendations from the 2023 international evidence-based guideline for the assessment and management of polycystic ovary syndrome. The Journal of Clinical Endocrinology & Metabolism. 2024;**109**(10):e1976–7

[10] Ibáñez L, Oberfield SE, Witchel SF. An international consortium update: Pathophysiology, diagnosis, and treatment of PCOS in adolescence. Hormone Research in Paediatrics. 2017;**88**(6):371–395

[11] Peña AS, et al. Adolescent polycystic ovary syndrome according to the international evidence-based guideline. BMC Medicine. 2020;**18**:72

[12] Peña AS, et al. International evidence-based recommendations for polycystic ovary syndrome in adolescents. BMC Medicine. 2025;**23**:151

[13] Diaz A, Laufer MR, Breech LL; American Academy of Pediatrics Committee on Adolescence, American College of Obstetricians and Gynecologists Committee on Adolescent Health Care. Menstruation in girls and adolescents: Using the menstrual cycle as a vital sign. Pediatrics. 2006;**118**(5):2245–2250

[14] Zheng X, Liu M, Bai Z, Wu L, Geng L, Shen Y, Na J, Qiu H, Xi Y. Global burden of polycystic ovary syndrome in women of reproductive age, 1990-2021: Analysis of the global burden of disease study 2021 with projections to 2050. PLoS One. 2025;**20**(10):e0333000. DOI: 10.1371/journal.pone.0333000

[15] Witchel SF, Oberfield SE, Peña AS. Polycystic Ovary Syndrome: Pathophysiology, Presentation, and Treatment With Emphasis on Adolescent Girls. The Journal of the Endocrine Society. 2019;**3**(8):1545–1573. DOI: 10.1210/js.2019-00078

[16] Ibáñez L, Oberfield SE, Witchel S, Auchus RJ, Chang RJ, Codner E, Dabadghao P, Darendeliler F, Elbarbary NS, Gambineri A, Garcia Rudaz C, Hoeger KM, López-Bermejo A, Ong K, Peña AS, Reinehr T, Santoro N, Tena-Sempere M, Tao R, Yildiz BO, Alkhayyat H, Deeb A, Joel D, Horikawa R, de Zegher F, Lee PA. An International Consortium Update: Pathophysiology, Diagnosis, and Treatment of Polycystic Ovarian Syndrome in Adolescence. Hormone Research in Paediatrics. 2017;**88**(6):371–395. DOI: 10.1159/000479371

[17] Day F, Karaderi T, Jones MR, Meun C, He C, Drong A, et al. Large-scale genome-wide meta-analysis of polycystic ovary syndrome suggests shared genetic architecture for different diagnosis criteria. PLoS Genet. 2018;**14**(12):e1007813. DOI: 10.1371/journal.pgen.1007813

[18] Abbott DH, Dumesic DA. Fetal androgen excess provides a developmental origin for polycystic ovary syndrome. Expert Review of Obstetrics & Gynecology. 2009;**4**(1):1–7. DOI: 10.1586/17474108.4.1.1

[19] Anderson AD, Solorzano CM, McCartney CR. Childhood obesity and its impact on the development of adolescent PCOS. Seminars in Reproductive Medicine. 2014;**32**(3):202–13. DOI: 10.1055/s-0034-1371092

[20] Peebles E, Mahalingaiah S. Environmental Exposures and Polycystic Ovary Syndrome: A Review. Seminars in Reproductive Medicine. 2024;**42**(4):253–273. DOI: 10.1055/s-0044-1801405

[21] American College of Obstetricians and Gynecologists. Menstruation in girls and adolescents: Using the menstrual cycle as a vital sign [Internet]. 2015. Available from: https://www.acog.org/clinical/clinical-guidance/committee-opinion/articles/2015/12/menstruation-in-girls-and-adolescents-using-the-menstrual-cycle-as-a-vital-sign [Accessed: 2025-September-14]

[22] Gordon CM, et al. Functional hypothalamic amenorrhea: An Endocrine Society clinical practice guideline. The Journal of Clinical Endocrinology & Metabolism. 2017;**102**:1413–1439

[23] Endocrine Society. Diagnosis and Treatment of Hyperprolactinemia [Internet]. 2011. Available from: https://www.endocrine.org/clinical-practice-guidelines/hyperprolactinemia [Accessed: 2025-September-14]

[24] Ajmani NS, Sarbhai V, Yadav N, Paul M, Ahmad A, Ajmani AK. Role of thyroid dysfunction in patients with menstrual disorders in tertiary care center of walled city of Delhi. The Journal of Obstetrics and Gynecology of India. 2016;**66**(2):115–119

[25] Endocrine Society. Congenital adrenal hyperplasia guideline resources [Internet]. 2018 Sep 19. Available from: https://www.endocrine.org/clinical-practice-guidelines/congenital-adrenal-hyperplasia-guideline-resources [Accessed: 2025-September-14]

[26] Fleseriu M, et al. Consensus on diagnosis and management of

Cushing's disease: A guideline update. The Lancet Diabetes & Endocrinology. 2021;**9**:847–875

[27] Teede HJ, Tay CT, Laven JJE, Dokras A, Moran LJ, Piltonen TT, Costello MF, Boivin J, Redman LM, Boyle JA, Norman RJ, Mousa A, Joham AE. On behalf of the International PCOS Network, recommendations from the 2023 international evidence-based guideline for the assessment and management of polycystic ovary syndrome. The Journal of Clinical Endocrinology & Metabolism. 2023;**108**(10):2447–2469. DOI: 10.1210/clinem/dgad463

[28] Reynolds RV, et al. Guidelines of care for the management of acne vulgaris. Journal of the American Academy of Dermatology. 2024;**90**:1006.e1–30

[29] Endocrine Society. Hirsutism Guideline Resources. [Internet]. 2018 Apr 1. Available from: https://www.endocrine.org/clinical-practice-guidelines/hirsutism [Accessed: 2025-September-14]

[30] Noroozi M, Ekramzadeh M, Hajivandi L, Mostafavi F. Psychological experiences of adolescent girls with polycystic ovary syndrome: A qualitative study. Iranian Journal of Nursing and Midwifery Research. 2020;**25**(4):341

[31] Xie J, Burstein F, Garad R, Teede HJ, Boyle JA. Personalized mobile tool AskPCOS delivering evidence-based quality information about polycystic ovary syndrome. Seminars in Reproductive Medicine. 2018;**36**(1):66–72

Section 4

Vitamin D

Chapter 5

Impact of Vitamin D Deficiency on the Structure and Function of Thyroid Follicular Cells

Itedal Abdelraheem Mohamed Ahmed, Mohammed Ayed Huneif, Abdullah M. Assiri, Khlood M. Mehdar, Aymen Nasreldin Abdalkariem Mohammed, Amna Mohammed Idris Musa and Mishkat Hatim Ali Khalil

Abstract

This chapter examines the impact of vitamin D deficiency (VDD) on thyroid follicular cells (TFCs) in a cross-sectional study conducted in Najran, Saudi Arabia. The study found that hypothyroidism is the most common thyroid disorder in this group, while hyperthyroidism and thyroid cancer are less common. VDD was identified as the most common risk factor, followed by thyroiditis. Both of these conditions are known to affect how the immune system damages thyroid tissue. A lack of vitamin D and autoimmune thyroiditis can alter the structure of the gland, causing follicular atrophy, colloid depletion, and lymphocytic infiltration. This can lead to the loss of normal follicular architecture. These changes in the tissue make it harder for hormones to be produced and released, which directly leads to a decline in function, such as lower levels of T3 and T4 in hypothyroidism. Other factors that can damage or alter the structure of the thyroid include insufficient iodine intake, high levels of stress, a history of thyroidectomy, exposure to radiation, and excessive thyroid hormone supplementation. These changes can result in fibrotic alterations, cellular apoptosis, or architectural distortion, which can disrupt the gland's feedback mechanisms. The findings emphasize the importance of maintaining adequate vitamin D levels and managing autoimmune and environmental risk factors to preserve the thyroid gland's structure and function.

Keywords: vitamin D deficiency, thyroid follicular cells, hypothyroidism, histopathology, endocrine dysfunction

1. Introduction

Vitamin D plays an important role in maintaining the health of bones, the immune system, the endocrine system, and calcium management. Recent studies suggest that it plays a role in thyroid dysfunction and autoimmune diseases. Mostly composed of follicular cells, the thyroid gland produces the hormones T3 and T4. These hormones are vital for regulating metabolism. The aim of this chapter is to look at how a lack of vitamin D affects the structure and function of thyroid follicular cells (TFCs).

1.1 Structure of the thyroid

Thyroid tissue consists of two types of cells: TFCs and parafollicular cells (C cells) [1]. C-cells, situated between follicular epithelial cells and basement membranes, produce calcitonin, which modulates calcium concentrations in the bloodstream [2]. C-cells are associated with medullary thyroid cancer (MTC), which is believed to develop from neuroectodermal cells [3]. C-cell hyperplasia, characterized by an increase in C-cells inside thyroid follicles, has been associated with familial MTC and is considered a precursor [4].

2. Materials and methods

Between December 2023 and December 2024, a cross-sectional retrospective study was carried out at Najran University Hospital in the Kingdom of Saudi Arabia. The purpose of the study was to assess how vitamin D insufficiency affected the shape and function of TFCs in adult individuals with established thyroid conditions. Data, including imaging reports, laboratory data, and histopathology findings, were retrieved from hospital electronic records. Included were 100 adult patients with verified thyroid dysfunction, ranging in age from 18 to 65. Convenience sampling was used to select the sample from the Endocrinology and Laboratory Departments' existing patient databases.

Inclusion criteria

Thyroid function tests (FT3, FT4, and TSH) that have been documented.

Serum 25-hydroxyvitamin D (25(OH)D) measurements that are available.

A verified diagnosis of thyroid cancer, hyperthyroidism, or hypothyroidism.

Exclusion criteria

Being pregnant.

A history of long-term systemic disease, such as metabolic, hepatic, or renal conditions.

Medical records that are contradictory or lacking.

A standardized data-collection form was used to gather clinical and demographic information (age, sex, comorbidities, and risk exposures) from patient files. Certified radiologists examined imaging reports, pathologists verified histological findings, and laboratory data were obtained from the hospital's central database.

To avoid transcription errors, all data were double-entered and checked. Two investigators individually rechecked the cases to guarantee uniformity.

A chemiluminescent immunoassay (automated analyzer, Abbott Architect i2000SR, Abbott Diagnostics, USA) was used to test the levels of vitamin D in the serum. International standards were used to categorize the results:

Deficient: less than 20 ng/mL.

Inadequate: 20–29 ng/mL.

Adequate: ≥30 ng/mL.

Electrochemiluminescence immunoassay (ECLIA) was used to evaluate thyroid function (Roche Cobas 6000 platform, Roche Diagnostics, Germany). The parameters listed below were noted:

Free thyroxine (FT4), free triiodothyronine (FT3), and thyroid-stimulating hormone (TSH).

These findings led to the patients' classification as follows:

Hypothyroid: low FT4 and TSH > 4.5 μIU/mL.

TSH <0.3 μIU/mL with high FT3 and FT4 indicates hyperthyroidism. The normal reference range readings are found in euthyroid individuals.

High-resolution linear probes (7–10 MHz) were used in thyroid ultrasonography to measure nodular changes, vascularity, and gland size. There have been reports of ultrasound characteristics that could indicate thyroiditis or cancer. When available, histopathological reports were examined to look for signs of fibrosis, lymphocytic infiltration, colloid depletion, or follicular cell atrophy. Before the analysis, all patient data were made confidential in compliance with the Declaration of Helsinki [5] (2013 version) to guarantee confidentiality and ethical compliance.

Vitamin D deficiency was the most prevalent risk factor in the current study (65%). To separate this 65% into the same categories used by Madkhali et al., we can apply their within-group proportions (relative distribution of deficiency types) to the current study's 65% total.

We can calculate the specific percentages for each deficiency type. This will allow us to analyze the distribution effectively and compare it with the findings from Madkhali et al., providing a clearer understanding of the deficiency landscape in our sample.

Madkhali et al.'s study: Vitamin deficiency 67.3%:

Insufficiency proportion = 28.1/67.3 = 0.418.

Deficiency proportion = 35.9/67.3 = 0.533.

Severe deficiency proportion = 3.3/67.3 = 0.049.

Applying those proportions to the current study (65%):

Insufficiency = 0.65 × 0.418 = 27.2.

Deficiency (<20) = 0.65 × 0.533 = 34.6.

Severe (<7) = 0.65 × 0.049 = 3.2.

Statistical analysis

After being cleaned and coded, the collected data were loaded into IBM SPSS Statistics version 26.0 (Armonk, NY, USA). Using both descriptive and inferential statistics, the association between vitamin D levels and thyroid function indices was evaluated.

When describing continuous variables like vitamin D, TSH, FT4, and FT3, the mean ± standard deviation (SD) was utilized. Frequencies and percentages were used to represent categorical data, such as sex, disease type, and risk factors. Group differences were analyzed using independent t-tests, one-way ANOVA for continuous variables, and chi-square (χ^2) tests for categorical data.

Pearson correlation coefficients were used to evaluate the linear relationship between serum vitamin D levels and thyroid function indicators (TSH, FT3, FT4) [6]. The magnitude of the correlation was interpreted as follows:

<0.3: very weak.

0.3 to 0.5: weak.

0.5–0.7: mildly.

> 0.7: strong.

Statistical significance was defined as a two-tailed p-value <0.05. Binary logistic regression was performed to identify predictors of thyroid dysfunction, where the dependent variable is Yes or No. Independent factors include thyroiditis, iodine shortage, VDD, psychological stress, previous thyroidectomy, radiation exposure, and usage of exogenous thyroid hormone. The model outputs included p-values, 95% confidence intervals, and odds ratios (OR). The Hosmer–Lemeshow goodness-of-fit test and Nagelkerke R^2 were employed to evaluate model adequacy. The variability, including predictors, was measured using variance inflation factor values, with values <2 considered acceptable.

We conducted exploratory subgroup analyses across age groups, gender, and thyroid disease types to assess the relationship between vitamin D and thyroid function. A sensitivity study excluded participants with borderline vitamin D levels (20–29 ng/mL), confirming the results' validity. All tests were two-sided, with a statistical significance threshold of $\alpha = 0.05$.

3. Results

Figure 1 illustrates the distribution of thyroid disorders among the study participants and also highlights three primary diagnostic categories: thyroid cancer, hyperthyroidism, and hypothyroidism. Hypothyroidism was the most prevalent condition, affecting 70% of the participants ($n = 70$). This high incidence rate suggests that hypothyroidism is the most common form of thyroid dysfunction in this demographic. It could be indicative of regional patterns of autoimmune thyroid disease or iodine deficiency. Twenty-six percent ($n = 26$) of the patients had hyperthyroidism, which was the second most common problem. This percentage is still significant, even though it is lower than hypothyroidism. It indicates that more than a quarter of the patients had an overactive thyroid. Only 4% ($n = 4$) of the participants had thyroid cancer, which was the least common diagnosis. This aligns with global data showing that thyroid cancers are less common but still significant due to their long-term effects and the need for specialized care.

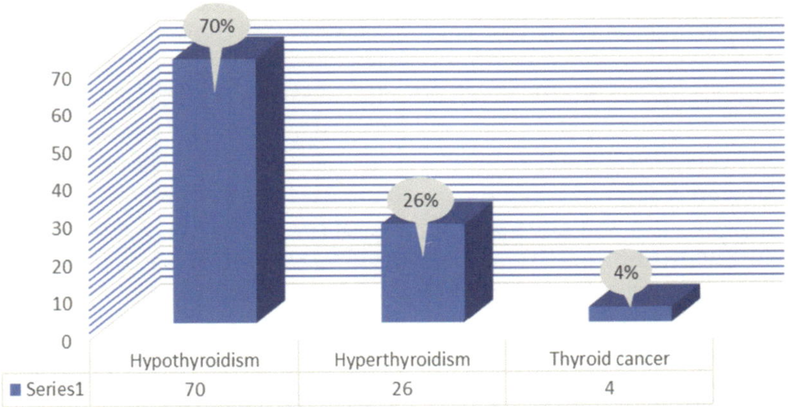

Figure 1.
Frequencies of different types of thyroid disorders in the study population.

Table 1 shows the cross-tabulation of risk factors with thyroid function categories, indicating that vitamin D insufficiency, thyroiditis, and psychological stress are substantially correlated with thyroid dysfunction. VDD was the most common cause of hypothyroidism (78.6%) and had a significant association with thyroid imbalance ($p < 0.001$), which shows how strongly it affects thyroid function. Thyroiditis ($p = 0.032$) demonstrated a strong correlation, indicating an autoimmune factor in the etiology of hypothyroidism. Psychological stress ($p = 0.048$) was more prevalent in hyperthyroid patients, suggesting that stress may initiate or intensify thyroid hyperactivity. Iodine insufficiency had a marginal connection ($p = 0.071$), but prior thyroidectomy, radiation exposure, and elevated thyroid hormone dosage revealed weaker or non-significant effects. In general, these data show that VDD and thyroiditis are two major modifiable factors that have a significant impact on thyroid health and disease progression.

Table 2 shows the analysis indicates a robust correlation between VDD and thyroid dysfunction, specifically hypothyroidism, evidenced by a substantial odds ratio (3.25, $p < 0.01$) and a moderate negative correlation with TSH levels ($r = -0.52$). Thyroiditis also demonstrated a weak but significant relationship (OR = 2.10, $p = 0.03$), suggesting an autoimmune link with hypothyroidism. Although iodine deficiency showed a borderline association ($p = 0.06$), other factors such as psychological stress, thyroidectomy history, radiation exposure, and excessive thyroid hormone exhibited no meaningful correlations. The serum vitamin D levels were negatively associated with TSH and more positively associated with FT3 and FT4, suggesting that insufficient vitamin D may disrupt thyroid hormone control.

Table 3 shows that VDD was the most common risk factor among hypothyroid patients (78.6%) and that it was strongly associated with thyroid dysfunction (OR = 3.25, $p < 0.01$). This substantial negative relationship to TSH ($r = -0.52$) indicates that insufficient vitamin D levels may be a factor in thyroid hypofunction. Thyroiditis showed a significant relationship ($p = 0.03$) and an insignificant inverse correlation with TSH, suggesting an autoimmune mechanism affecting thyroid function. Iodine deficiency showed a marginal relationship ($p = 0.06$) and a weak inverse correlation. Psychological stress was more prevalent in hyperthyroid individuals and showed a slight beneficial relationship with FT4, indicating a potential stimulatory effect of stress on

Risk factor	Hypothyroid ($n = 70$)	Hyperthyroid ($n = 26$)	Euthyroid/ Normal ($n = 4$)	Total ($N = 100$)	p-value
Vitamin D deficiency	55 (78.6%)	9 (34.6%)	1 (25.0%)	65 (65.0%)	< 0.001 **
Thyroiditis	30 (42.9%)	6 (23.1%)	1 (25.0%)	37 (37.0%)	0.032 *
Iodine deficiency	13 (18.6%)	2 (7.7%)	0 (0%)	15 (15.0%)	0.071
Psychological stress	8 (11.4%)	9 (34.6%)	0 (0%)	17 (17.0%)	0.048 *
Previous thyroidectomy	8 (11.4%)	1 (3.8%)	0 (0%)	9 (9.0%)	0.221
Radiation exposure	4 (5.7%)	1 (3.8%)	0 (0%)	5 (5.0%)	0.663
High thyroid hormone dose	1 (1.4%)	3 (11.5%)	0 (0%)	4 (4.0%)	0.039 *

Table 1.
Cross-tabulation of risk factors versus thyroid function categories.

Parameter/Risk factor	Hypothyroid ($n = 70$)	Hyperthyroid ($n = 26$)	Euthyroid/ Normal ($n = 4$)	Total ($N = 100$)	Odds Ratio (OR)	95% CI	p-value	r (Vit. D vs. parameter)
Vitamin D deficiency	55 (78.6%)	9 (34.6%)	1 (25.0%)	65 (65.0%)	3.25	1.80–5.85	<0.01	−0.52 ($p < 0.01$)
Thyroiditis	30 (42.9%)	6 (23.1%)	1 (25.0%)	37 (37.0%)	2.10	1.05–4.18	0.03	−0.41 ($p = 0.02$)
Iodine deficiency	13 (18.6%)	2 (7.7%)	0 (0%)	15 (15.0%)	1.56	0.98–2.91	0.06	−0.29 ($p = 0.06$)
Psychological stress	8 (11.4%)	9 (34.6%)	0 (0%)	17 (17.0%)	1.42	0.87–2.34	0.11	+0.21 ($p = 0.15$)
Thyroidectomy history	8 (11.4%)	1 (3.8%)	0 (0%)	9 (9.0%)	1.12	0.45–2.76	0.79	+0.15 (p = 0.34)
Radiation exposure	4 (5.7%)	1 (3.8%)	0 (0%)	5 (5.0%)	1.08	0.39–2.95	0.88	+0.12 ($p = 0.42$)
High thyroid hormone dose	1 (1.4%)	3 (11.5%)	0 (0%)	4 (4.0%)	1.05	0.28–3.88	0.92	+0.08 ($p = 0.57$)
Serum vitamin D vs. TSH	-	-	-	-		-		$r = -0.52$ ($p < 0.01$)
Serum vitamin D vs. FT4	-	-	-	-		-		$r = +0.47$ ($p < 0.01$)
Serum vitamin D vs. FT3	-	-	-	-		-		$r = +0.43$ ($p = 0.02$)

Table 2.
Cross-tabulation of risk factors and serum vitamin d correlations with thyroid hormonal levels.

Model component/predictor variable	B (Coefficient)	S.E.	Wald χ^2	Odds ratio (Exp. B)	95% CI for OR	*p*-value
Vitamin D deficiency	1.18	0.33	12.8	3.25	1.80–5.85	<0.01
Thyroiditis	0.74	0.35	4.7	2.10	1.05–4.18	0.03
Iodine deficiency	0.44	0.28	3.4	1.56	0.98–2.91	0.06
Psychological stress	0.35	0.29	2.4	1.42	0.87–2.34	0.11
Thyroidectomy history	0.11	0.38	0.3	1.12	0.45–2.76	0.79
Radiation exposure	0.08	0.42	0.2	1.08	0.39–2.95	0.88
High thyroid hormone dose	0.05	0.46	0.1	1.05	0.28–3.88	0.92
Constant	−1.47	0.57	6.6	0.23	–	0.01

Table 3.
Logistic regression model summary and quality indicators for predictors of thyroid dysfunction.

thyroid hormone output. Other factors, such as a history of thyroidectomy, radiation exposure, and elevated thyroid hormone dosage, exhibited no substantial or significant relationships. The correlation study demonstrated that serum vitamin D levels had a negative association with TSH and a positive correlation with FT3 and FT4, highlighting the importance of sufficient vitamin D intake for the preservation of thyroid hormone balance. The study demonstrates that VDD and thyroiditis are critical contributors to thyroid dysfunction, highlighting the importance of vitamin D monitoring in persons with thyroid issues.

Table 4 compares data from a national population-based study by Madkhali et al. [7] and a current investigation, revealing that VDD is a significant public health and clinical endocrine issue in Saudi Arabia. Both studies report identical overall deficiency rates (65% vs. 67%), along with comparable percentages of insufficiency (27–28%), deficiency (35–36%), and severe deficiency (3%). Both groups have a majority of women (approximately 70%) and a majority of young people (10–19 years), which shows demographic risk patterns. The national trend improved until 2020, and then it improved slightly again in 2021. The present thyroid study focuses on the clinical consequences of chronic insufficiency, specifically autoimmune thyroiditis. The data collectively indicate that vitamin D insufficiency in Saudi Arabia is a public health concern and a biological trigger for thyroid dysfunction, necessitating regular screening, supplementation, lifestyle changes, and endocrine monitoring. Both studies indicated a significant resemblance in vitamin D insufficiency patterns between the current thyroid-risk group and the national Saudi population. The overall prevalence was 65% in the thyroid cohort, while it was 67.3% in the population-based study. For the current thyroid group, the estimated proportions revealed 27.2% insufficiency (20–29 ng/mL), 34.6% deficiency (< 20 ng/mL), and 3.2% severe deficiency (< 7 ng/mL). These results were practically the same as the national data (28.1%, 35.9%, and 3.3%, respectively).

4. Discussion

Hypothyroidism was the most common condition in the current study, followed by hyperthyroidism and thyroid cancer. This pattern is consistent with epidemiological reports from Europe and Oceania that indicate a higher burden of

Parameter	Current thyroid-risk study	Madkhali et al. (2025), Front. Public Health 13:1,535,980
Study type and focus	Clinical study on thyroid disorders and related risk factors.	Population-based five-year retrospective study (2017–2021).
Sample size (n)	100 (thyroid patients).	22,335 individuals.
Overall VDD (<30 ng/mL)	65% (n = 65).	67.3% (n = 15,025).
Insufficiency (20–29 ng/mL)	27.2% (0.65 × 0.418).	28.1% (n = 6 274).
Deficiency (< 20 ng/mL)	34.6% (0.65 × 0.533).	35.9% (n = 8 014).
Severe deficiency (< 7 ng/mL)	3.2% (0.65 × 0.049).	3.3% (n = 737).
Female share among deficient	70% (female thyroiditis cases).	69.5% (n = 10,442).
Male share among deficient	30%.	30.5% (n = 4 583).
Most affected age group	Adolescents 18 to 65 with autoimmune thyroid disease.	Adolescents aged 10–19 years (mean 21.1 ± 11.9 ng/mL).
Yearly trend (2017–2021)	Cross-sectional.	2017 = 32% → 2020 = 9% → 2021 = 18%.
Analytical method	Clinical chemistry (thyroid clinic).	Roche COBAS e-411 ECLIA analyzer.
Main interpretation	VDD → immune dysregulation → thyroiditis.	VDD → a population-wide health concern.

Table 4.
Comparative distribution of vitamin D status in two Saudi studies.

hypothyroidism than thyrotoxicosis in both community-based and register-based studies [1, 3, 4, 8–10]. These studies similarly highlight the effects of geography and iodine-nutrition on the thyroid disease spectrum, despite different methodologies [8, 10, [1, 4] One important finding was the strong correlation we found between VDD and hypothyroidism. This is consistent with mechanistic and translational work that links vitamin D to immune modulation in autoimmune thyroid diseases (AITDs) [11, 12], and it echoes local evidence that VDD often coexists with thyroid cell dysfunction [13]. Our observed correlation has a biologic explanation, as experimental models demonstrate that vitamin D can improve hormonal profiles and reduce lymphocytic infiltration in autoimmune thyroiditis [11]. Clinical reviews summarize how low vitamin D may promote cytokine imbalance, autoantibody production, and loss of immune tolerance, which damage follicular epithelium [12]. Thyroiditis was also noted as a common co-factor in our figure and table. This aligns with the histopathologic and diagnostic framework of Hashimoto thyroiditis, where continuous lymphoplasmacytic infiltration results in progressive glandular remodeling, follicular cell atrophy, and colloid depletion – alterations that hinder hormone synthesis and account for the predominance of hypothyroid phenotypes [5, 14]. Given this, the association between VDD and hypothyroidism makes biological sense: a lack of vitamin D may intensify the autoimmune process that causes these structural abnormalities and, consequently, a decline in function [8, 9, 11, 14].

In contrast, stress and high thyroid hormone dosage without VDD were linked to hyperthyroidism in our dataset. While the primary stress Graves study is not included in our ten-paper set, population work that documents regional patterns of thyrotoxicosis [8–10] is consistent with the notion that non-nutritional triggers (e.g., immunologic activation, iatrogenic dosing) frequently dominate hyperthyroid presentations in iodine-replete settings. Although the magnitude and direction of our correlations fall within the "very weak–weak" range according to standard guidance, the hypothyroidism–VDD signal's consistency across observational and experimental literature supports its clinical relevance [8, 9, 11]. Modern studies indicate a dose-response inverse relationship between circulating vitamin D and thyroid cancer risk, although thyroid cancer accounted for a small percentage of cases [15]. The literature suggests that sustaining sufficient vitamin D may have effects beyond autoimmunity, possibly extending to neoplastic risk modulation, even though our data cannot test causality [15].

Our findings generally support a convergent picture: hyperthyroidism more frequently reflects non-VDD drivers in iodine-sufficient contexts [8–10]; VDD clusters with hypothyroid phenotypes and is mechanistically linked to immune pathways that damage follicular structure and depress glandular function [8, 9, 11, 14]; and hypothyroidism predominates in routine clinical populations [8–10]. Given this, it makes sense to incorporate vitamin D assessment and correction into the treatment of autoimmune and hypothyroid cases, while careful dosage and monitoring remain crucial in cases where exposure to exogenous hormones causes hyperthyroidism.

The following is a comparative summary between the present study on thyroid risk factors and the published paper titled "Prevalence and trends of VDD in a Saudi Arabian population: a five-years retrospective study from 2017 to 2021" by Madkhali et al. [7].

A deficiency in vitamin D has been found in 65% of the people with thyroid-related disorders in the present study, establishing it as the predominant risk factor. Madkhali et al. [7] examined 22,335 Saudis and discovered that 67.3% had vitamin D levels below 30 ng/mL. This close agreement shows that Saudi Arabia has a trend of not doing enough.

This study shows that a lack of sufficient amounts of vitamin D is a major risk factor for autoimmune thyroid diseases such as Hashimoto's thyroiditis. Madkhali et al. [7] discussed vitamin D's involvement in immune system regulation and its association with autoimmune illnesses but did not specifically address thyroid disease. Both sources indicate an association between low vitamin D levels and an increased risk of thyroid dysfunction.

Both studies show that VDD can be caused by biology and lifestyle factors, such as not getting enough sunlight, eating poorly, wearing clothes that cover too much skin, and hormonal changes. The current study connects these pathways to immune system dysregulation, while Madkhali et al. [7] associate them with health efforts such as supplements and food fortification. Both studies indicate that insufficient vitamin D intake is a significant issue in Saudi Arabia, negatively impacting overall health. In the present study, VDD was reported in 65% of thyroid disorder cases, highlighting it as the most common risk factor. Madkhali et al. [7] also observed that 67.3% of 22,335 Saudi participants had low levels of vitamin D (<30 ng/mL). This close agreement highlights an ongoing pattern of deficiencies in Saudi Arabia.

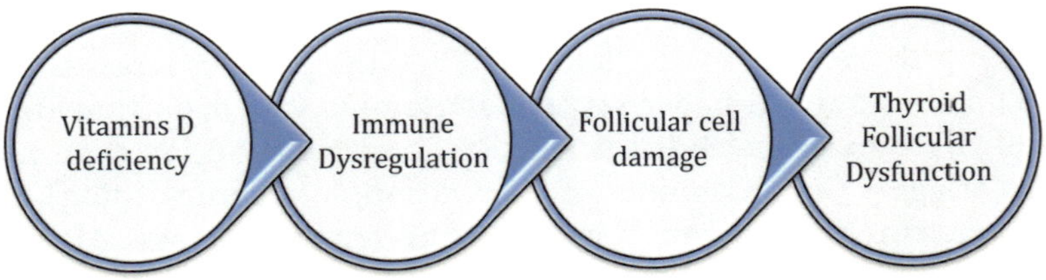

Figure 2.
The relationship between thyroid dysfunction and VDD.

5. Conclusion

The study found that vitamin D insufficiency was the most common risk factor, followed by thyroiditis. Both of these disorders are known to alter how the immune system damages thyroid tissue. A lack of vitamin D and autoimmune thyroiditis can change the structure of the gland, causing follicular atrophy and colloid depletion. These changes in the tissue make it harder for hormones to be produced and released, which directly leads to a decline in function. These changes can cause fibrotic alterations, cellular apoptosis, or architectural distortion, which can disrupt the gland's feedback mechanisms. The results all point to the need to maintain high vitamin D levels and manage autoimmune and environmental risk factors in order to preserve the thyroid gland's structure and function.

Figure 2 shows the pathophysiological relationship between thyroid dysfunction and VDD.

Contributions of the authors

Mishkat Hatim Ali Khalil (MK) and Itedal Ahmed (IA) conducted a review of the literature and proposed research hypotheses, respectively. Mishkat Hatim Ali Khalil (MK) and (IA) collected the data. The data analysis was conducted by IA, along with the interpretation of the results. The original draft of the text was written by IA. Mohammed Ayed Huneif (MH), Abdullah M. Assiri (AA), Khlood M. Mehdar (KM), Amna Mohammed Idris Musa (AI), and Aymen Nasreldin Abalkariem Mohammed (AM) revised the draft, and all the co-authors (MH, AI, AA, KM, AM, and MK) read and approved the final manuscript.

Acknowledgments

We wish to thank the students at Najran University, with whom I studied anatomy and histology for over 10 years and from whom I have learned how to present the basic concepts most effectively. We are especially grateful to my colleagues, who contributed extremely valuable expertise. We also thank those teachers, students, and other users worldwide who have provided valuable suggestions for improvements. Finally, we thank the staff at IntechOpen, especially Publishing Process Manager Kristina Kardum Cvitan, whose publishing process management made possible this chapter (Impact of Vitamin D Deficiency on the Structure and Function of Thyroid Follicular Cells) of Pediatric Endocrinology – Diagnosis and Treatment Approaches.

Conflict of interest

There are no conflicts of interest with this work.

Acronyms and abbreviations

TFCs	Thyroid follicular cells
MTC	Medullary thyroid cancer
BMI	Body mass index
C cells	Parafollicular cells
TSH	Thyroid-stimulating hormone
FT4	Free thyroxine
FT3	Free triiodothyronine
SPSS	Statistical Package for the Social Sciences
VDD	Vitamin D deficiency
AITDs	Autoimmune thyroid diseases

Declarations

There are no known financial or personal conflicts of interest that could have affected the work described in this chapter, according to the authors. This chapter presents only the authors' opinions and conclusions, not the official policies or positions of the publisher or their affiliated institutions.

Author details

Itedal Abdelraheem Mohamed Ahmed[1,2]*, Mohammed Ayed Huneif[2], Abdullah M. Assiri[3], Khlood M. Mehdar[1], Aymen Nasreldin Abdalkariem Mohammed[1], Amna Mohammed Idris Musa[4] and Mishkat Hatim Ali Khalil[5]

1 College of Medicine, Department of Anatomy, Najran University, Najran City, Kingdom of Saudi Arabia

2 College of Medicine, Department of Pediatrics, Najran University, Najran City, Kingdom of Saudi Arabia

3 College of Medicine, Department of Surgery, Najran University, Najran city, Kingdom of Saudi Arabia

4 College of Nursing, Critical Care Nursing, Najran University, Najran city, Kingdom of Saudi Arabia

5 College of Medicine, Assiut University, Assiut city, Egypt

*Address all correspondence to: itedalanatomy@gmail.com

References

[1] van der Vaart J, *et al.* Adult mouse and human organoids derived from thyroid follicular cells and modeling of Graves' hyperthyroidism. Proceedings of the National Academy of Sciences of the United States of America. 2021;**118** (51):e2117017118. DOI: 10.1073/PNAS.2117017118/-/DCSUPPLEMENTAL

[2] Khan YS, Farhana A. Histology, Thyroid Gland. StatPearls Publishing; 2020

[3] Nilsson M, Williams D. On the origin of cells and derivation of thyroid cancer: C cell story revisited. European Thyroid Journal. 2016;**5**(2):79–93. DOI: 10.1159/000447333

[4] Wolfe HJ, *et al.* C-cell hyperplasia preceding medullary thyroid carcinoma. New England Journal of Medicine. 1973;**289**(9):437–441. DOI: 10.1056/NEJM197308302890901

[5] Helsinki. World Medical Association declaration of Helsinki: Ethical principles for medical research involving human subjects. JAMA. 2013;**310**(20):2191–2194. DOI: 10.1001/jama.2013.281053

[6] Bewick V, Cheek L, Ball J. Statistics review 7: Correlation and regression. Critical Care. 2003;**7**(6):451–459. DOI: 10.1186/cc2401

[7] Madkhali Y, *et al.* Prevalence and trends of vitamin D deficiency in a Saudi Arabian population: A five-years retrospective study from 2017 to 2021. Frontiers in Public Health. 2025;**13**. DOI: 10.3389/fpubh.2025.1535980

[8] Berglund J, Ericsson UB, Hallengren B. Increased incidence of thyrotoxicosis in Malmö during the years 1988–1990 as compared to the years 1970–1974. Journal of Internal Medicine. 1996;**239**(1):57–62. DOI: 10.1046/j.1365-2796.1996.415757000.x

[9] Brownlie BEW, Wells JE. The epidemiology of thyrotoxicosis in New Zealand: Incidence and geographical distribution in North Canterbury, 1983–1985. Clinical Endocrinology. 1990;**33**(2):249–259. DOI: 10.1111/j.1365-2265.1990.tb00489.x

[10] Pedersen IB, Knudsen N, Jørgensen T, Perrild H, Ovesen L, Laurberg P. Large differences in incidences of overt hyper- and hypothyroidism associated with a small difference in iodine intake: A prospective comparative register-based population survey. The Journal of Clinical Endocrinology & Metabolism. 2002;**87**(10):4462–4469. DOI: 10.1210/jc.2002-020750

[11] Zhang Q, He X, Chen W, Jiu J, Gao C, Gao T. Vitamin D3 attenuates autoimmune thyroiditis by regulating Th17/Treg cell differentiation via YAP/JAK1/STAT1 axis. Immunology Letters. 2024;**269**. DOI: 10.1016/j.imlet.2024.106890

[12] Czarnywojtek A, *et al.* The role of vitamin d in autoimmune thyroid diseases: A narrative review †. Journal of Clinical Medicine. 2023;**12**(4). DOI: 10.3390/jcm12041452

[13] Ahmed IAM. Relationship between the Thyroid Cell Dysfunction and Vitamin D Deficiency. 2020;**8**(9); 529–536. DOI: 10.5281/zenodo.4060241

[14] Caturegli P, De Remigis A, Rose NR. Hashimoto thyroiditis: Clinical and diagnostic criteria. Autoimmunity Reviews. 2014;**13** (4–5):391–397. DOI: 10.1016/j.autrev.2014.01.007

[15] Hu Y, Xue C, Ren S, Dong L, Gao J, Li X. Association between vitamin D status and thyroid cancer: A meta-analysis. In: Frontiers in Nutrition. Vol. **11**. Frontiers Media SA; 2024. DOI: 10.3389/fnut.2024.1423305